THE INSULIN PUMP THERAPY BOOK

INSIGHTS FROM THE EXPERTS

EDITED BY LINDA FREDRICKSON,
MA, RN, CDE

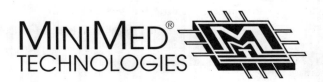

Sof-set™, Quick Release™, Polyfin™, SportGuard™, and ShowerPak™ are trademarks of MiniMed, Inc.

Copyright © 1995 by MiniMed Inc.
First Published in Los Angeles, California
Manufactured in the United States of America

Produced by the Professional Education Department of MiniMed Technologies

Editor: Linda Fredrickson, MA, RN, CDE

For more information, write the Professional Education Department
MiniMed Technologies
12744 San Fernando Rd.
Sylmar, CA 91342.

ISBN 0-9647837-0-3

Library of Congress Catalog Card Number: 95-78723

Typesetting, Design and Cover Origination by GreyZone Creative Services, Saugus CA
Printed by All Valley Printing, Chatsworth, CA

FOREWORD

Over the past 15 years, there has been increasing interest in intensive management of diabetes with insulin pump therapy. The unequivocal demonstration by the Diabetes Control and Complications Trial in 1993 that intensive management can dramatically reduce the risks for development or progression of retinopathy, nephropathy, and neuropathy in insulin-dependent diabetes mellitus has greatly heightened the interest in and need for such therapy. Although blood glucose can be lowered to near-normal levels by using multiple daily injections of various combinations of intermediate- or long-acting insulin with regular insulin, such an approach has certain impediments. Most frustrating of these is the unpredictable absorption of insulin from its various sites of injection and under varying circumstances, which leads to a mismatch between insulin availability and glucose entry into the bloodstream from either endogenous or dietary sources.

Insulin pump therapy circumvents and minimizes this and other problems, and therefore, offers state-of-the-art management for people wishing to have optimum control over their diabetes. To implement insulin pump therapy properly, however, requires a firm knowledge of its principles and the details of its day-to-day use. Given this challenge, physicians, health care professionals, and people who wish to control their diabetes with insulin pump therapy are fortunate to have new tools, like this book, to help them.

As an endocrinologist, diabetes researcher, and physician who treats people with diabetes, I am pleased that this book has been written. The authors are well-recognized as diabetes specialists with worldwide reputations as insulin pump experts. The book deals with all aspects of pump therapy in a straightforward and understandable, yet comprehensive, manner. The fundamentals of pump management are accurately captured in each chapter. *The Insulin Pump Therapy Book: Insights from the Experts* represents a significant contribution to enhancing diabetes care and should be read by all persons setting out to maximize the care of diabetes through pump therapy.

Saul Genuth, MD
Professor of Medicine, Case Western Reserve University
Chief of Endocrinology, Mt. Sinai Health Care Systems
Cleveland, Ohio

PREFACE

Since selling our first insulin pump in 1983, MiniMed has been dedicated to educating physicians and diabetes educators who prescribe pump therapy, as well as the individuals who use our pumps. To date, thousands of health care professionals have participated in academic symposia sponsored by MiniMed, and our pump therapy educational materials for laypersons and professionals are used the world over.

This book grew out of discussions among the prominent diabetologists and pump experts who lead our symposia series. They expressed a need for a complete, authoritative resource book on insulin pump therapy that would be addressed to the health care professional, and that might also be useful for pump users who wish to gain maximum benefits from pump therapy.

It is our hope that *The Insulin Pump Therapy Book: Insights from the Experts* will fulfill this need by communicating the knowledge and experience of some of the foremost authorities on insulin pump therapy. We hope, also, that it serves to further establish insulin pump therapy as a cost-effective mode of intensive diabetes management that not only facilitates normalized blood glucose, but also makes it feasible for people living with diabetes to experience the most normal lifestyle possible.

For the pump user, this book is intended only as a guide, and should not be construed as professional health care advice. Insulin requirements and treatment protocols differ significantly from one person to the next and must be developed individually under the guidance of a professional health care team.

As always, we welcome your comments and suggestions. This book will be updated periodically to incorporate reader feedback, new research findings, and technology advances.

Linda Fredrickson, MA, RN, CDE
Director, Professional Education and Clinical Services
Phone: 818-362-5958 or 800-933-3322 • FAX 818-364-0968
e-mail: LFRED@ix.netcom.com

"For the first time in my life, I know that I will die from something other than diabetes."

Carl Aframe, MiniMed Pump User
Diabetes Forecast, *August 1994*

To all the dedicated and courageous participants in the Diabetes Control and Complications Trial. Without your commitment, we might never have known the difference that intensive diabetes management can make.

ACKNOWLEDGEMENTS

We express our great thanks to all who have provided us with clinical information, readily answered our questions, reviewed chapters, loaned research data, and edited manuscript.Special thanks to Mary Specker Stone of Health Care Communications, who, along with her assistant, Sharon Jones, edited each manuscript from the various chapter authors; and to Christy G. Stevenson, MiniMed's Professional Education Manager, who developed the cover concept and helped in many other ways to make this book possible.

IN PARTICULAR, WE THANK:

Jo Ann Ahern, RN, MA, CDE

Bernadette D'Almedia, RN

Edward Etkind, MD

Ruth Farkas-Hirsch, MS, RN, CDE

Stanley Feld, MD, FACE

Charleen Freeman, RN, CDE

John Galloway, MD

Saul Genuth, MD

Paula Harper, RN, CDE

Susan F. Hill, MS, RD, CDE

Edward S. Horton, MD

Denise Ingegneri, MS, RD, CDE

Paul S. Jellinger, MD, FACE

Donna L. Jornsay, RN, BSN, CPNP, CDE

Lois Jovanovic-Peterson, MD

Lexy Justus, RD, CDE

Alan O. Marcus, MD, FACP

Jorge H. Mestman, MD

Stig K. Pramming, MD

Lisa E. Rafkin-Mervis, MS, RD, CDE

Chris Sadler, MA, CDE

TABLE OF CONTENTS

CHAPTER AUTHOR

I

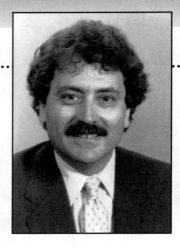

JAY S. SKYLER, MD

Dr. Skyler is Professor of Medicine, Pediatrics, and Psychology at the University of Miami in Miami, Florida. One of the most respected endocrinologists of our time, Dr. Skyler has written and edited numerous articles, book chapters, and editorials and has lectured internationally for over 20 years on diabetes-related topics, and specifically on the importance of intensive diabetes management. Dr. Skyler is study chair of the nationwide Diabetes Prevention Trial for type I diabetes (DPT-1) sponsored by the National Institutes of Health. He is also past president of the American Diabetes Association (ADA) and served as founding Editor-in-Chief of the ADA professional journal, *Diabetes Care*.

INTRODUCTION

"The Quest for Normoglycemia." So Robert Tattersall titled his recent lucid historical review of the more than 70-year struggle by diabetologists and their patients with diabetes to maintain glycemic status as close to normal as safely possible (1). This goal was initially recommended in 1923, shortly after the discovery of insulin. It was also articulated in 1993 by the DCCT investigators, as they concluded their heroic study that clearly and unequivocally demonstrated the benefits of meticulous control in reducing the risks of the chronic complications of diabetes (2). Yet, although the basic goals may be the same, much has evolved in our therapeutic arsenal to help physicians and people with diabetes wrestle with the problem of correcting the hyperglycemic state that characterizes type I diabetes mellitus. One of the critical advances in these efforts has been the development of continuous subcutaneous insulin infusion (CSII) as a clinical strategy.

EVOLUTION OF CSII

The idea of continuous insulin delivery first emerged in the early 1960s. At that time, Dr. Arnold Kadish of Los Angeles fashioned a device (Figure 1) that would permit such insulin delivery. As can be seen, the device was so cumbersome that its widespread use was not practical. In the late 1970s there was further evolution of the concept that insulin replacement ideally should be provided in a physiologic manner, in which there was replacement of both basal insulin secretion and prandial incremental insulin secretion. In several parts of the world, a number of investigators attempted this with intravenous insulin delivery. These included Gerard Slama and his colleagues in France, Dieter Hepp's group

IN THIS CHAPTER

Evolution of CSII

Investigating the Value of Near-Normoglycemia

CSII in the DCCT

Advantages of CSII

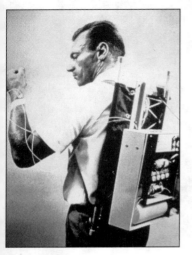

Figure 1

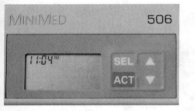

Figure 2

in Germany, and Saul Genuth and coworkers in the United States (3-5). After this, attempts were made to deliver such physiologic insulin replacement subcutaneously.

The first reports of experience with portable pumps for CSII came in 1978 from Harry Keen, John Pickup, and their colleagues at Guy's Hospital in London (6). This was followed in early 1979 by a widely read report from William Tamborlane, Philip Felig and coworkers at Yale (7). These early studies demonstrated that CSII, when used together with self-monitoring of blood glucose (SMBG) in a program of what came to be known as "Intensive Insulin Therapy" made it possible to achieve plasma glucose levels near the normal range (8). Thus, "intensive therapy" emerged into the clinical arena, with the demonstrated feasibility of achieving near-normal glycemic control.

Early insulin pumps were relatively bulky (up to 400 grams in weight, and as large as 18.3 x 7.3 x 6.4 centimeters). They required that batteries be recharged or changed on a frequent basis, and that insulin be diluted. With time, the pumps have become much smaller (Figure 2), compatible with commercial insulin preparations, associated with long-lived batteries (two months), and easier to use. Multiple safety alarms are now built-in. Today's pumps permit the programming of multiple basal rates, profiling of boluses, suspension or temporary rate programming of insulin delivery during exercise, memory display of historical insulin delivery, and softened catheters which do not require that an insertion needle be left in place. The recent introduction of "quick release" infusion set technology permits the pump user to easily disconnect from the infusion tubing during such activities as showering, swimming, shopping (with multiple changes of clothes), and sexual intimacy. All of these advances have combined to make CSII a viable, safe therapy to offer people with diabetes in the 1990s.

INVESTIGATING THE VALUE OF NEAR-NORMOGLYCEMIA

By the time (the late 1970s) that CSII was being first explored as a treatment modality for type I diabetes, there had been other important developments as well:

- Evidence supporting a relationship between glycemic control and the chronic complications of diabetes had accumulated from epidemiologic studies, non-randomized clinic studies, and studies in animal models.
- A reliable quantitative method of assessing glycemic control, i.e., HbA_{1c}, had been developed, thus permitting quantification and verification of the effect of intervention.
- Reliable quantitative methods of assessing endpoints related to diabetic complications had been developed to a degree sufficient for use in multicenter clinical trials.

All of these developments coalesced and led to the design and conduct of prospective, randomized intervention studies to test the impact of meticulous glycemic control on diabetic complications.

A number of small prospective, randomized studies were initiated, including those conducted under the auspices of the Steno Memorial Hospital in Gentofte, Denmark; the Kroc Foundation Oligo Multicenter Study in the US and UK; the Aker Hospital in Oslo, Norway; the Aahrus (Denmark) Study; the Stockholm Diabetes Intervention Study; and others. Of these studies, most (Steno, Kroc, Aker, Aahrus) used CSII to assure adequate and reproducible insulin delivery. Meanwhile, in the United States, to try to answer the question with sufficient statistical power to draw a relatively firm conclusion, the DCCT (Diabetes Control and Complications Trial) was designed. In 1993, after 9000 patient years of observation, the DCCT reported its results (2). It conclusively demonstrated the beneficial effects and impact of effective glycemic control on chronic complications of type I diabetes and forever changed the way diabetes must be treated.

The DCCT involved randomizing participants at 29 centers to either "conventional" treatment or "intensive" treatment. "Intensive" treatment consisted of CSII or multiple daily insulin injections (MDI, three to four injections per day), with the therapy choice left to the investigator and participant; SMBG three to four times daily, with additional specified samples, including a weekly overnight sample; meticulous attention to diet; and monthly visits to the treating clinic. "Conventional" treatments consisted of no more than two daily insulin injections; urine glucose monitoring or SMBG no more than twice daily; periodic diet review; and clinic visits every two to three months.

The DCCT had been planned to have statistical power to detect a 33.5 percent treatment effect for diabetic retinopathy. Many observers had hoped for at best a 40 percent reduction in event rates in the intensive therapy group versus the conventional therapy group. The results dramatically exceeded anyone's wildest expectations: the intensive therapy group demonstrated a 70 percent reduction in risk of retinopathy progression, a 40 to 54 percent reduction in incidence of nephropathy, and a 64 percent reduction in incidence of neuropathy. Yet, these beneficial effects of intensive therapy were not without associated risks. Severe hypoglycemia, defined as those episodes requiring assistance of another person to recover, was increased threefold in the intensive therapy group, including a threefold increased risk of coma or seizures consequent to hypoglycemia. Importantly, 55 percent of severe hypoglycemic episodes occurred during sleep.

The DCCT conclusively demonstrated the beneficial effects and impact of effective glycemic control on chronic complications of type I diabetes and forever changed the way diabetes must be treated.

CSII IN THE DCCT

CSII was widely used in the DCCT (9). Fully 59 percent of intensively-treated subjects tried CSII for some period of time, and 34 percent used CSII on an ongoing, long-term basis. Forty-two (42) percent of subjects used CSII during 1992, the last full year of the study (Figure 3). CSII subjects achieved 0.2 percent to 0.4 percent lower HbA_{1c} levels than MDI subjects. This level of control was associated with a slightly higher rate of hypoglycemic events resulting in coma or seizure, but not a greater incidence of total episodes of severe hypoglycemia. The increase in coma/seizure was accounted for by a greater number of such events per subject experiencing them, as there was no difference in the proportion of subjects having such events. Even then, the event rate for coma or seizure was only 18 episodes per 100 patient years of follow-up, or 1 episode every 5.6 patient years of follow-up. Infections at sites of catheters used for CSII occurred at a rate of 12 episodes per 100 patient years of follow-up, or 1 episode every 8.3 patient years of follow-up.

Figure 3

Percent of intensively treated patients in the DCCT using CSII, by study year.

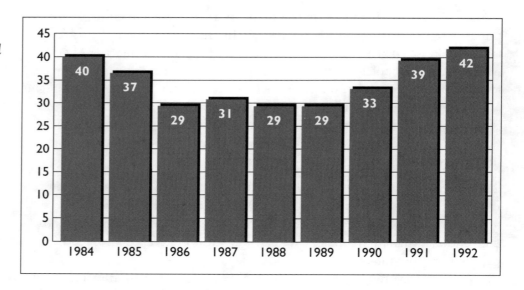

During their presentation of results, the DCCT investigators stated that CSII facilitated nocturnal glycemic control and provided greater flexibility in lifestyle. They also asserted that intensive therapy is best implemented in centers with the requisite nursing, dietary, behavioral, and clinical expertise to ensure safe and effective therapy. And, they indicated that they had used flexibility and "unrestrained creativity" in the design of intensive therapy programs, individualizing them to meet the needs of the patient and making ongoing adaptations aimed at achieving the therapeutic targets.

ADVANTAGES AND UTILITY OF CSII

So, where does that leave us, in the aftermath of the DCCT? The American Diabetes Association has revised its standards of care to recommend intensive therapy, with a goal of near-normal glycemic control, in most persons with type I diabetes (10). In the implementation of intensive therapy, CSII offers several potential advantages. These include pharmacokinetic advantages, which derive from: (a) CSII using only rapid-acting regular insulin, thus having more reproducible insulin absorption; (b) using only one body region for insulin delivery, thus avoiding interregional variation of insulin absorption; and (c) the absence of insulin accumulation in a subcutaneous depot, thus reducing the risk of mobilizing that depot with exercise, and thereby lessening the likelihood of exercise-related hypoglycemia. Another advantage derives from the programmability of CSII, both surrounding meals and overnight. Mealtime programmability offers pump users greater flexibility of lifestyle, and overnight programmability facilitates nocturnal glycemic control to aid in both avoiding nocturnal hypoglycemia and preventing the dawn phenomenon.

Because of these advantages, it is my bias that CSII should be considered by all persons with type I diabetes. CSII must always be used in the context of a complete program of intensive therapy. Therefore, my practice is to implement the other elements of intensive therapy first, thus allowing the person to distinguish the impact of CSII per se. As a consequence, CSII is used in selected, motivated individuals who desire a more normal lifestyle without sabotaging glycemic control. Another important use is in those people who require reproducible insulin delivery, e.g., those who fail to recognize hypoglycemic symptoms and/or to spontaneously recover from hypoglycemia. In the past, these may have been considered persons in whom CSII should be avoided. However, it is now evident that in these persons CSII permits reproducible insulin delivery with less risk of hypoglycemia, provided glycemic targets are set higher.

IN CLOSING

In the chapters that follow, CSII is discussed extensively. These chapters have been prepared by an experienced group of experts who provide practical insights into implementation of CSII therapy. This book should prove useful to health care professionals in counseling individuals who are considering CSII and in managing those using intensive therapy with CSII. It may also prove useful for people with diabetes who are in the process of integrating CSII into their lives.

REFERENCES

1. Tattersall RB. The quest for normoglycemia: a historical perspective. *Diabetologia.* 1994;11:618-635.

2. The Diabetes Control and Complications Trial Research Group. The effect of intensive treatment of diabetes on the development and progression of long-term complications in insulin-dependent diabetes mellitus. *N Engl J Med* 1993;329:683-689.

3. Slama G, Hautecouverture M, Assan R, Tchobroutsky G. One to five days of continuous intravenous insulin infusion on seven diabetic patients. *Diabetes* 1974;23:732-738.

4. Hepp KD, Renner R, von Funcke HJ, Mehnert H, Haerten R and Kresse H. Glucose homeostasis under continuous intravenous insulin therapy in diabetics. *Horm Metab Res* 1977;Suppl 7:72-76.

5. Genuth S, Martin P. Control of hyperglycemia in adult diabetics by pulsed insulin delivery. *Diabetes* 1977;26:571-581.

6. Pickup JC, Keen H, Parsons JA, Alberti KGMM. Continuous subcutaneous insulin infusion: an approach to achieving normoglycemia. *Br Med J* 1978;1:204-207.

7. Tamborlane WV, Sherwin RS, Genel M, Felig P. Reduction to normal of plasma glucose in juvenile diabetes by subcutaneous administration of insulin with a portable infusion pump. *N Engl J Med* 1979;300:573-578.

8. Schade DS, Santiago JV, Skyler JS, Rizza R. *Intensive Insulin Therapy.* Princeton, NJ: Excerpta Medica, 1983.

9. Diabetes Control and Complications Trial Research Group. Implementation of treatment protocols in the Diabetes Control and Complications Trial. *Diabetes Care* 1995;18:361-376.

10. American Diabetes Association. Standards of medical care for patients with diabetes mellitus. *Diabetes Care* 1994;17:616-623.

CHAPTER AUTHORS

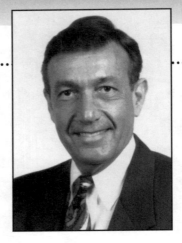

PHILIP RASKIN, MD

Dr. Raskin is a professor of medicine in the Department of Internal Medicine at the University of Texas Southwestern Medical Center in Dallas, Texas. He has been the editor of *Journal of Diabetes and Its Complications* since 1992 and was formerly the editor of *Clinical Diabetes*. Dr. Raskin serves as the Director of the University Diabetes Treatment Center and Diabetes Outpatient Clinic at Parkland Memorial Hospital in Dallas. He has worked with Suzanne Strowig for more than a decade providing intensive management with insulin pumps to hundreds of people with diabetes.

SUZANNE M. STROWIG, MSN, RN, CDE

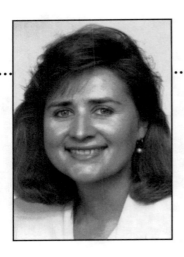

Ms. Strowig, a faculty associate in the Department of Internal Medicine at the University of Texas Southwestern Medical Center, is a diabetes clinical nurse specialist and consultant in both diabetes education and clinical management. She has written many articles on pump therapy and lectures throughout the country on the Diabetes Control and Complications Trial (DCCT), intensive diabetes management, and insulin pump therapy. Ms. Strowig was the DCCT Trial Coordinator at the University of Texas throughout the study's nine-year term. Ms. Strowig has worked with Dr. Raskin for more than a decade specializing in the intensive management of diabetes using insulin pumps. In addition to her other speaking engagements and writing activities, she has been an instructor on insulin pump therapy with the Advanced Studies Institute for Diabetes Education since 1992.

Benefits of Insulin Pump Therapy

2

Continuous subcutaneous insulin infusion (CSII) offers the most physiologic mode of insulin delivery currently available and is a valuable component of intensive treatment in people with IDDM and selected individuals with NIDDM. As an alternative to multiple daily injections (MDI), CSII offers a number of significant benefits, including more predictable insulin absorption and reduced risk for severe hypoglycemia. Most importantly, CSII provides an effective means to attain near-normal blood glucose levels, which have been associated with improved pregnancy outcomes and reduced risk for long-term diabetic complications. In addition, CSII permits people who use insulin to live a more normal lifestyle, giving them the capability to readily adjust their dosage to meet both known and unanticipated changes in need.

CSII: A TOOL FOR NORMALIZING BLOOD GLUCOSE LEVELS

Early studies demonstrated the effectiveness of pump therapy in helping people with diabetes achieve near-normal glycemia (1-3). These and other studies also helped to provide a better understanding of the relationship between hyperglycemia and diabetic complications. Normalized blood glucose was linked to:

- Improved plasma glucagon profiles (4).
- Improved lipid and lipoprotein levels (5).
- Improved motor nerve conduction velocities (6).
- Stabilization of background retinopathy and incipient nephropathy (7, 8).
- Reduced risk for microvascular complications, as measured by skeletal muscle capillary basement membrane thickness (9).

IN THIS CHAPTER

CSII as a Tool

Value of Careful Glycemic Control

Current Standard of Care: Near–Normal Glycemia

Benefits of Insulin Pump Therapy

Longer-term studies further documented the effectiveness of CSII-based intensive management in safely normalizing blood glucose levels (10-14).

In the nine-year Diabetes Control and Complications Trial (DCCT), participants using an intensive treatment program to maintain near-normal blood glucose levels had an overall 60 percent reduction in the risk for microvascular complications compared to participants on conventional injection therapy (14). Those in the intensive therapy group followed a comprehensive program of care, including physiologic insulin administration using either CSII or multiple daily injection.

Overall, the DCCT intensive treatment group had a mean HbA_{1c} of 7.2 percent, whereas the conventionally treated group maintained a significantly higher mean HbA_{1c} of 8.9 percent. Within the intensive treatment group, the mean glycosylated hemoglobin was 0.2 percent to 0.4 percent lower in the subgroup predominantly treated with the insulin pump for five years (n = 124), as compared with those using predominantly multiple daily injection (n=284) (15).

THE VALUE OF CAREFUL GLYCEMIC CONTROL

The value of careful glycemic control in reducing the risk for microvascular and macrovascular diabetic complications has been clearly demonstrated by the DCCT and two other major longitudinal studies: the eight-year Wisconsin Epidemiologic Study of Diabetic Retinopathy (WESDR) (16), and the eight-year Stockholm Diabetes Intervention Study (SDIS) (17).

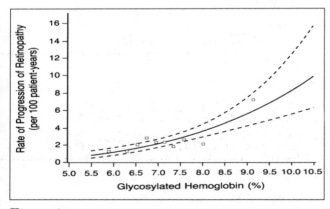

Figure 1
Risk of sustained progression of retinopathy in DCCT patients receiving intensive therapy, according to their mean glycosylated hemoglobin values during the trial. Dashed lines are 95% confidence limits. Reprinted with permission (14).

Reduced development and progression of retinopathy

In the DCCT, intensive therapy reduced the risk for the development of retinopathy by 76 percent relative to participants treated with conventional injection therapy. In participants with existing retinopathy, intensive treatment slowed its progression by 54 percent and reduced the development of proliferative retinopathy by 47 percent.

Secondary analysis of the DCCT data revealed a continuous decrease in the rate of progression of retinopathy with decreasing glycemia: every 10 percent decrease (e.g., from 10 percent to 9 percent or from 9 percent to 8.1 percent) in HbA_{1c} was associated with an approximately 40 percent reduction in the risk of developing retinopathy (18).

In the WESDR study, investigators found a similarly strong and consistent association between hyper-

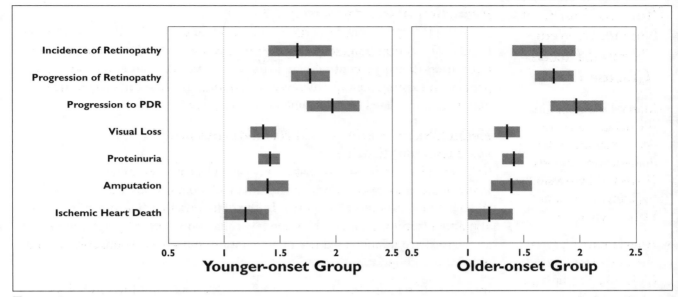

Figure 2

The effect on risk of development of complications by a one percent increase in glycosylated hemoglobin at baseline in participants of the Wisconsin Epidemiologic Study of Diabetic Retinopathy (16). Graphs show risk ratio and 95% confidence limits. Reprinted with permission

glycemia and the incidence and progression of retinopathy in participants with both insulin-dependent and non-insulin-dependent diabetes (16). Glycosylated hemoglobin at baseline was found to be the most important risk factor for the incidence and progression of retinopathy, regardless of the type or duration of diabetes.

Investigators in the Stockholm study estimated threshold glycemic levels for protection against retinopathy. They found that participants with mild retinopathy at baseline who maintained a mean HbA_{1c} of less than 7 percent (normal range, 3.9–5.7 percent) for five years did not tend to develop serious retinopathy or experience deterioration in visual acuity by study year 7.5 (17). While near-normoglycemia did not prevent the progression of more advanced nonproliferative retinopathy to proliferative retinopathy, it did tend to protect visual acuity following laser photocoagulation.

Reduction in risk for nephropathy

In the DCCT, intensive therapy reduced the occurrence of gross proteinuria by 54 percent (14). Klein and colleagues in the WESDR study also observed a strong relationship between hyperglycemia and development of gross proteinuria (16). An HbA_{1c} of less than 9 percent was found by Reichard et al to protect against development of nephropathy at 7.5 years in participants with either normal albumin excretion or microalbuminuria at baseline (17).

Proven Benefits of Normal or Near-Normal Blood Glucose Levels

- Marked reduction in the danger of acute decompensation due to diabetic ketoacidosis (DKA) or hyperosmolar hyperglycemic non-ketotic syndrome.

- Alleviation of hyperglycemic symptoms (polyuria, polydipsia, fatigue, weight loss with polyphagia, blurred vision, and vaginitis or balanitis).

- Greatly decreased risks for development or progression of diabetic retinopathy, nephropathy, and neuropathy.

- Reduction in atherogenicity of lipid profile in persons with lipoprotein abnormalities.

Reduction in risk for neuropathy

Intensive therapy reduced the risk for clinical neuropathy by 60 percent in the DCCT. The Stockholm group observed that participants who maintained an HbA_{1c} less than 7 percent seldom developed neuropathy, and that some participants with existing neuropathy reversed it during the 7.5-year study if they maintained this level of blood glucose control (17).

Reduction in risk for cardiovascular and peripheral vascular complications

Klein found a significant association between glycemia and mortality from ischemic heart disease in both participants with younger-onset diabetes and those with older-onset disease (16). In the older-onset participants, there was also a significant association between glycemia and stroke. Hyperglycemia was associated with an increased risk of amputation in both the younger-onset and older-onset groups.

Intensive therapy in the DCCT reduced the development of hypercholesterolemia by 34 percent and the risk for overall cardiovascular and peripheral vascular events by 41 percent (14).

Near-term benefits of tight control

In addition to these long-term benefits of near-normal blood glucose control, there are both short-term and mid-term benefits. The importance of euglycemia prior to and during the pregnancies of diabetic women is well-known (see Chapter 13, *Pump Therapy in Preconception and Pregnancy*). In the short term, people with diabetes who maintain stable control at near-normal glycemic levels report that they feel and function better (19).

THE CURRENT STANDARD OF CARE: NEAR-NORMAL GLYCEMIA

Because of its proven value in reducing the risk of long-term diabetic complications as well as the acute risks and symptoms of the disease, "Treatment aimed at lowering blood glucose levels to or near normal in all patients is mandated..." according to the American Diabetes Association (20). As a component of intensive therapy in persons with IDDM and some with NIDDM the ADA recommends "physiologically based insulin regimens," using CSII or multiple daily injections.

ADDITIONAL BENEFITS OF INSULIN PUMP THERAPY

Insulin pump therapy offers a number of important benefits beyond those of improved control of blood glucose. Among these are:

More physiologic mode of insulin delivery

Insulin delivery from a pump more closely mimics that from a healthy pancreas: it combines a continuous background level of insulin (basal delivery) with bolus

The Dawn Phenomenon and CSII

The dawn phenomenon, experienced by approximately 80 percent of people with insulin-dependent diabetes, is characterized by a pronounced early-morning rise in blood glucose levels and insulin requirements. It is thought to be due to accelerated glucose production in the dawn hours, coupled with an early morning rise in serum cortisol and growth hormone (21).

Koivisto et al demonstrated that the dawn rise in glucose production and plasma glucose could be prevented by increasing insulin delivery during the dawn hours (21). As shown in Figure 3, continuous infusion with a constant rate of insulin allowed plasma glucose levels to rise during the dawn hours; however, when the infusion rate was stepped up by 50 percent, no increase in plasma glucose was seen, similar to the control (non-diabetic) group's profile.

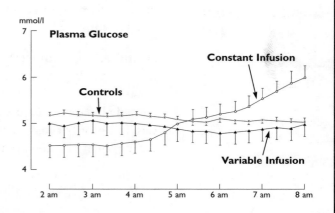

Figure 3

Changes in plasma glucose levels in healthy controls and in participants with type I diabetes during CSII with constant or increased infusion rate (21). Reprinted with permission.

doses at mealtime and in response to elevated blood glucose levels. The capability to control basal and bolus doses independently of each other allows the pump user flexibility in dealing with both anticipated and unanticipated changes in insulin need. For example, pump users who experience the dawn phenomenon are able to program an increase in the basal rate during the dawn hours. Premeal bolus doses can be given at the time the meal is consumed, permitting precise dosage adjustment according to the content of the meal and any planned exercise after the meal. If a meal is skipped or delayed, the basal dose maintains glycemic control.

More predictable insulin absorption

Intermediate- and long-acting insulins do not provide a constant basal insulin supply due to their highly variable absorption, which ranges from 10 percent to 52 percent of the injected daily dose (22). Variable insulin absorption is responsible for up to 80 percent of the day-to-day fluctuation in blood glucose concentrations in persons using injection-based therapy (23). In contrast, regular insulin delivered by an insulin pump shows far more predictable absorption, varying by less than 2.8 percent from the administered 24-hour dose (22). CSII therefore provides the greatest day-to-day reproducibility in insulin availability, and the least unexpected fluctuation in glycemic control.

Another pharmacokinetic advantage of the insulin pump is that plasma insulin peaks appear within 30 to 90 minutes after administration of meal bolus doses, which is sufficient to maintain near-normal blood levels following meals (22). Predictable postprandial peaks are seldom seen with conventionally administered insulin (22).

Reduced risk for severe hypoglycemia
More stable blood glucose levels can be achieved with pump therapy, as discussed above, and therefore the risk of hypoglycemia is reduced. The pump's variable basal rate feature allows the pump user to match the insulin delivery rate to his or her insulin need, programming a lower delivery rate, for example, during the nighttime hours if nocturnal hypoglycemia tends to be a problem.

Pumps are particularly useful in avoiding overinsulinization in people who are highly sensitive to insulin; doses as small as 0.1 unit can be accurately delivered. Because there is only a minimal subcutaneous insulin depot with CSII, the risk of exercise-induced hypoglycemia is also reduced.

More normal lifestyle
CSII allows pump users to be fully in charge of their day-to-day diabetes care decisions and to live a more normal lifestyle than multiple daily injections would permit. Pump users can adjust insulin delivery in response to changes in schedule, activity level, meal times, and other events of daily life, without having to plan around timed insulin injections and periods of peak insulin action. In this regard, pump therapy is particularly well-suited for people who travel frequently, work variable shifts, or have erratic schedules or levels of physical exertion.

OUR EXPERIENCE WITH CSII-BASED INTENSIVE TREATMENT

As a DCCT investigational site, we have gained extensive experience with both MDI and CSII in intensive therapy regimens. We have observed that persons using CSII do measurably better than those using multiple daily injections, given the same amount of self-care effort. Many of our DCCT participants who were unable to achieve their blood glucose goals while using multiple daily injections were successful in safely attaining their goals when switched to an insulin pump. Based on our experience, we believe that the pharmacokinetics of CSII make it a superior mode of insulin delivery in intensive treatment.

Successful use of an insulin pump requires motivation on the part of the user, who must assume a high level of responsibility for the management of his or her disease. In addition to the usual demands of intensive therapy, including frequent self-monitoring of blood glucose, insulin adjustment, and dietary management, safe use of the insulin pump also requires that the user pay careful attention to pump and infusion set details (24). Ideally, CSII therapy should be supervised by a health care provider who is knowledgeable about intensive diabetes management and pump therapy, specifically, and who has access to specialists in the area of dietetics, diabetes education, and mental health.

Many of our DCCT participants who were unable to achieve their blood glucose goals while using multiple daily injections were successful in safely attaining their goals when switched to an insulin pump.

REFERENCES

1. Tamborlane WV, Sherwin RS, Genel M, Felig P. Reduction to normal of plasma glucose in juvenile diabetes by subcutaneous administration of insulin with a portable pump. *N Engl J Med* 1979;300:573-578.

2. Raskin P. Treatment of insulin-dependent diabetes with portable insulin infusion devices. *Med Clin North Am* 1982;66:1269-1283.

3. Mecklenburg RS, Benson EA, Benson JW, Blumenstein BA, Fredlund PN, Guinn TS, Metz RJ, Nielsen RL. Long-term metabolic control with insulin pump therapy. Report of experience with 127 patients. *N Engl J Med* 1985;313:465-468.

4. Raskin P, Unger RH. Hyperglucagonemia and its suppression. *N Engl J Med* 1978;299:433-436.

5. Dunn FL, Pietri A, Raskin P. Plasma lipid and lipoprotein levels with continuous subcutaneous insulin infusion in type I diabetes. *Ann Intern Med* 1981;95:426-431.

6. Pietri A, Ehle AL, Raskin P. Changes in nerve conduction velocity after six weeks of glucose regulation with portable insulin infusion pumps. *Diabetes* 1980;29:688-671.

7. Friberg TR, Rosenstock J, Sanborn G, Vaghefi A, Raskin P. The effect of long-term near normal glycemic control on mild diabetic retinopathy. *Ophthalmology* 1985;92:1051-1058.

8. The Kroc Collaborative Study Group. Blood glucose control and the evolution of diabetic retinopathy and albuminuria: a preliminary multicenter trial. *N Engl J Med* 1984;11:365-372.

9. Raskin P, Pietri A, Unger R, Shannon WA Jr. The effect of diabetic control on skeletal muscle capillary basement membrane width in patients with type I diabetes mellitus. *N Engl J Med* 1983;309:1546-1550.

10. Mecklenberg RS, Benson EA, Benson JW, Fredlund PN, Guinn T, Metz RJ, Nielsen R, Sannar C. Acute complications associated with insulin infusion pump therapy. Report of experience with 161 patients. *JAMA* 1984;252:3265-3269.

11. Eichner HL, Selam JL, Holleman CB, Worcester BR, Turner DS, Charles MA. Reduction of severe hypoglycemic events in type I (insulin dependent) diabetic patients using continuous subcutaneous insulin infusion. *Diabetes Res* 1988;8:189-193.

12. Chantelau E, Spraul M, Muhlhauser I, Gause R, Berger M. Long-term safety, efficacy and side-effects of continuous subcutaneous insulin infusion treatment for type 1 (insulin-dependent) diabetes mellitus: a one centre experience. *Diabetologia* 1989;32:421-426.

13. Wredling R, Lins P-E, Adamson U. Factors influencing the clinical outcome of continuous subcutaneous insulin infusion in routine practice. *Diabetes Res Clin Pract* 1993;19:59-67.

14. The Diabetes Control and Complications Trial Research Group. The effect of intensive treatment of diabetes on the development and progression of long-term complications in insulin-dependent diabetes mellitus. *N Engl J Med* 1993;329:977-986.

15. Diabetes Control and Complications Trial Research Group. Implementation of treatment protocols in the Diabetes Control and Complications Trial. *Diabetes Care* 1995:18:361-376.

16. Klein R. Hyperglycemia and microvascular and macrovascular disease in diabetes. *Diabetes Care* 1995;18:258-268.

17. Reichard P. Are there any glycemic thresholds for the serious microvascular diabetic complications? *J Diab Compl* 1995;9:25-30.

18. Lachin J. Relationship of glycemia to complications in the DCCT. Presented at the American Diabetes Association 54th annual meeting, New Orleans, LA, June 11, 1994.

19. Reichard P, Toomingas B, Rosenqvist U. Changes in conceptions and attitudes during five years of intensified conventional insulin treatment in the Stockholm diabetes intervention study (SDIS). *Diab Educ* 1994;20:503-508.

20. American Diabetes Association. Standards of medical care for patients with diabetes mellitus. *Diabetes Care* 1995;18(Suppl 1):8-15.

21. Koivisto VA, Yki-Jarvinen H, Helve E, Karonen S-L, Pelkonen R. Pathogenesis and prevention of the dawn phenomenon in diabetic patients treated with CSII. *Diabetes* 1986;35:78-82.

22. Lauritzen T, Pramming S, Deckert T, Binder C. Pharmacokinetics of continuous subcutaneous insulin infusion. *Diabetologia* 1983;24:326-329.

23. Binder C, Lauritzen T, Faber O, Pramming S. Insulin pharmacokinetics. *Diabetes Care* 1984;7:188-199.

24. Strowig SM. Initiation and management of insulin pump therapy. *Diabetes Educ* 1993;19:50-58.

CHAPTER AUTHOR

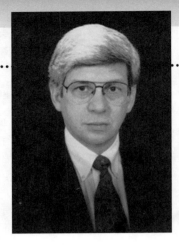

ROBERT J. TANENBERG, MD, FACP

Dr. Tanenberg is Clinical Associate Professor of Medicine at Georgetown University and Medical Director of the Diabetes Treatment Center at Washington Hospital Center in Washington, D.C. In his private endocrinology practice, he specializes in intensive management of patients with type I diabetes, in particular, adolescents, pregnant women, and adults with brittle diabetes. Dr. Tanenberg served as a consultant to the National Institutes of Health (NIH) for the Diabetes Control and Complications Trial. He has authored several articles and book chapters on diabetes management and lectures widely to both patients and health professionals on diabetes treatment and insulin pump therapy. Since 1990, Dr. Tanenberg has been a principal investigator for the MiniMed Implantable Pump Program.

CANDIDATE SELECTION

3

As a mode of insulin delivery for intensive diabetes therapy, continuous subcutaneous insulin infusion (CSII) offers an alternative to multiple daily insulin injections (MDI). CSII has been shown to be the optimal form of insulin delivery for highly motivated individuals who desire a greater level of participation in their diabetes self-care and for those who are unable to achieve good control or lead a normal life with multiple daily injection regimens.

Any program of intensive therapy places additional demands on insulin-using individuals and should not be undertaken by those who lack proper motivation, education, or medical support. CSII is no exception: it requires the same self-care behaviors used in MDI regimens, as well as additional behaviors relating to care of the infusion site and avoidance of rapid-onset diabetic ketoacidosis (DKA).

CSII PRESCRIBING GUIDELINES

A 1984 analysis by the Centers for Disease Control on the safety of pump use revealed that rates and causes of death were no different in individuals using pumps than in those using conventional insulin therapy (1). This report allayed early safety concerns surrounding pump use and set forth guidelines for the prescribing physician:

1. Set realistic goals for the level of glycemic control.

2. Actively encourage pump users to seek assistance in the event of intercurrent illness.

3. Pay careful attention to the pump user's motivation and compliance.

IN THIS CHAPTER

Prescribing Guidelines

Medical Indications

Realistic Expectations

Contraindications

This same study concluded that pump users must be willing, or already have demonstrated their ability, to:

- Monitor their own blood glucose levels regularly.
- Test urine for ketones during intercurrent illness.
- Maintain close contact with a friend or relative.
- Always have access to local medical care.
- Recognize warning signs of hypoglycemia and ketoacidosis.
- Understand, operate and maintain the insulin pump.
- Know the importance of good infusion techniques and catheter care.

Both the American Diabetes Association and the American Association of Diabetes Educators, in their position statements on CSII, emphasize that the person using CSII must assume substantial responsibility for decision-making and day-to-day care (2,3). The ideal insulin pump candidate, therefore, is an individual who has the knowledge and motivation to participate in the ultimate level of diabetes self-care (4). Often, this requires that he or she has had previous experience with intensive diabetes self-care, although pumps have been used successfully by individuals without such experience (5).

MEDICAL INDICATIONS FOR CSII

Improvement in Glycemic Control

The primary medical indication for insulin pump therapy is identical to that for other types of intensive diabetes therapy: to achieve better control of blood glucose levels and thereby reduce the risk for long-term diabetic complications. CSII, with its exclusive use of regular insulin, eliminates the unpredictable absorption of longer-acting insulins experienced by some individuals. This pharmacokinetic advantage makes CSII the preferred mode of insulin delivery for certain types of people attempting intensive control.

Insulin pump therapy can improve glycemic control in individuals with type I diabetes who are unable to achieve acceptable control on multiple daily injection regimens (6,7). Acceptable control is defined in advance by the health care provider and the person using insulin, and usually involves goals for target blood glucose levels, range of blood glucose levels (lability), and target HbA_{1c} levels.

CSII has also been used successfully in people with type II diabetes whose glycemia was poorly controlled with sulfonylurea drugs. In a study by A.M. Jennings and colleagues, 8 of 10 such participants treated with insulin pump therapy achieved a satisfactory level of glycemic control, whereas only 3 of 10 participants treated with conventional insulin injection therapy attained satisfactory control (8).

The primary medical indication for insulin pump therapy is... to achieve better control of blood glucose levels and thereby reduce the risk for long-term diabetic complications.

Hypoglycemia

As recently as a decade ago, insulin pump use was specifically contraindicated in individuals with recurrent, severe hypoglycemia or reduced hypoglycemic awareness. Now, however, CSII may be the insulin delivery method of first choice in people with a history of problems with hypoglycemia. Hirsch and colleagues used pump therapy in men and women with reduced hypoglycemic awareness to maintain glycemic control and reduce the incidence of severe hypoglycemia (9). In 205 study participants using pumps as part of a long-term intensive therapy regimen, Bode et al observed a sustained and significant reduction in the rate of severe hypoglycemia, accompanied by an equally significant reduction in HbA_{1c} levels (5).

Setting realistic target blood glucose levels for individuals on intensive therapy, including those using the insulin pump, is one of the most important factors in avoiding hypoglycemia (10). Both the Hirsch and Bode studies used higher target values than normoglycemic goals in pump users with a history of severe hypoglycemia or reduced hypoglycemic awareness (5,9). In contrast, severe hypoglycemia was problematic in the Diabetes Control and Complications Trial, where a normal HbA_{1c} was the target for all participants (11).

Pregnancy

Hyperglycemia in early pregnancy is known to be a major risk factor for congenital anomalies in infants born to mothers with diabetes. Intensive management of diabetes before conception and early in pregnancy has been shown to reduce the risk of congenital anomalies to the same level found in the non-diabetic population (12). CSII is a particularly useful method for intensification of insulin delivery in pregnant women with a history of hypoglycemia, wide blood glucose variations, or problems with the dawn phenomenon (12). It is also helpful in reducing hypoglycemia during morning sickness (13). Pregnant women should be encouraged to continue intensive therapy and pump use, if feasible, after pregnancy. (See Chapter 13, *Pump Therapy in Preconception and Pregnancy*).

Insulin Sensitivity

Extreme insulin sensitivity (total daily dose <20 U or <0.4 U/kg) is another indication for insulin pump therapy (10). The pump permits convenient administration of fractional insulin units (in 0.1 unit increments), a level of precision not available with injections.

Dawn Phenomenon

The insulin pump is the method of choice for delivering insulin in people with diabetes who experience fasting hyperglycemia due to the dawn phenomenon, or insulin waning in the early morning hours (4,10). A higher basal rate can be programmed for the early morning hours to counteract the rise in blood glucose.

CSII may be the insulin delivery method of first choice in people with a history of problems with hypoglycemia.

> *Insulin pump therapy can be viewed as the ultimate level of diabetes self-care, and successful preparation often involves a stepwise approach towards increasingly greater levels of self-care.*

Diabetic Complications

People with early diabetic complications (early neuropathy, nephropathy, or stable retinopathy) are often highly motivated to begin intensified therapy, as are kidney transplant recipients, in whom intensified therapy can help preserve the function of the new kidney (6). The pump offers a means of intensifying therapy, and thereby slowing the progression of complications, while allowing greater lifestyle flexibility (14).

Variable Work/Activity Schedules

People who have active, variable lifestyles are often the best candidates for insulin pump therapy (3,6,7,10). By providing the capability to alter basal rates (either temporarily or on a fixed schedule) and administer meal boluses precisely when needed, the insulin pump provides greater flexibility for people who work variable shifts, travel between time zones, and/or have erratic eating schedules due to meetings or other activities. The pump is also a good option for people whose activity level varies greatly during the day or from day to day, such as those who perform physical labor on a changing schedule.

PERSONAL FACTORS

Insulin pump therapy can be viewed as the ultimate level of diabetes self-care, and successful preparation often involves a stepwise approach towards increasingly greater levels of self-care (4,6). Several authors recommend that before changing to insulin pump therapy, individuals experience three to six months of intensified diabetes treatment (9,14). The best candidates for CSII therapy are people on multiple daily injections who have demonstrated their ability to perform and comply with diabetes self-care behaviors, including frequent self-monitoring of blood glucose (SMBG), insulin adjustment, and an understanding of dietary principles (e.g., use of an exchange system or carbohydrate counting) (3,7). However, pump therapy can be used successfully in motivated individuals who have limited experience in diabetes self-care when medically necessary (5). Additional candidate selection criteria are listed in Table 1.

Table 1

ATTRIBUTES AND ATTITUDES FOR SUCCESSFUL PUMP USE

Self-Motivation	The person must be willing to learn and accept responsibility for pump use, troubleshooting, and self-care behaviors. He or she must also agree to follow the recommended schedule for office visits, blood glucose reporting, etc.
Maturity	Insulin pumps have been used successfully in children, adolescents, adults, and seniors. Maturity is a more important determinant of pump success than age.
Acceptance of Diabetes	Wearing an insulin pump is a visible sign of diabetes. The pump cannot always be hidden during sports activities or intimate moments. Individuals who have not accepted their disease may feel uncomfortable relying on a pump for insulin, or making an outward "statement" that they have diabetes.
Intelligence/Ability to Solve Problems	The pump user must be capable of learning how to adjust insulin dosages according to blood glucose readings and to troubleshoot the pump, infusion set, and insulin dosage. Common sense and ability to follow a protocol are a MUST!
Demonstrated Ability to Perform Frequent (4+ Daily) SMBG	Frequent SMBG is an essential element of safe and effective pump therapy.

Expectations about CSII

It is important that pump candidates and their families have realistic expectations about pump therapy (Table 2). Unrealistic expectations can quickly lead to frustration and discontinuation of therapy, while realistic expectations can become the foundation for setting and attaining treatment goals.

Table 2

EXPECTATIONS ABOUT INSULIN PUMP THERAPY

Realistic	Unrealistic
I need to allow 3-6 months to adjust to pump therapy.	Pump therapy is easy–I'll adjust immediately.
I will feel better on pump therapy.	The insulin pump will cure my diabetes.
I will have more freedom with my diet and the timing of my meals.	I will have a totally free diet.
I will have better blood glucose control, less fluctuation in blood glucose levels, and less hyperglycemia.	I will have perfect blood glucose control with the pump. My postprandial blood glucose level will always be normal.
I will have to check my blood glucose levels 4 or more times every day.	I won't have to check my blood glucose levels regularly.

Adolescents are often more comfortable than adults with the technical aspects of pump therapy due to their experience with video games, VCRs, and computers.

Age

Pumps have been successfully used in children and adolescents. One study found that children with newly diagnosed diabetes achieved better metabolic control with insulin pump therapy than with conventional therapy (15). Bode and colleagues observed a marked decrease in the incidence of DKA in pump-treated adolescents whose previous poor control had been the result of erratic insulin dosing (written communication 1994). Other investigators have also observed improved control in adolescents treated with insulin pump therapy (16, 17). Adolescents are often more comfortable than adults with the technical aspects of pump therapy due to their experience with video games, VCRs, and computers. They also may benefit more from the flexibility in diet and lifestyle afforded by pump therapy, and by the reduced physical restriction in comparison to conventional injection therapy (16). Some young people, however, may choose to discontinue pump use during certain activities (contact sports, for example) or longer periods of seasonal activities (e.g., summer vacation). Maintaining insulin injection skills is therefore important. School personnel need to know that a child is wearing an insulin pump, and, as with injection therapy, the school nurse should receive written instructions from parents or health care professionals regarding hypoglycemia management.

Elderly individuals may be good candidates for insulin pump therapy as long as they are motivated, have no physical handicaps that prevent them from proper-ly programming the pump or inserting the catheter, and are free of end-stage diabetic complications.

Social and Psychological Factors

Use of an insulin pump requires psychological stability and positive support from close friends and family. Manipulative psychological behavior or over-dependency on a partner for diabetes care are contraindications to pump use (9, 18). If a health care provider is unsure of an individual's social or psychological status, further evaluation by a social worker or psychologist is recommended.

Psychological issues related to pump use include (19):

- *Privacy*: wearing an insulin pump may provoke questions, making it hard to remain private about one's illness.
- *Body image*: some single people are concerned about wearing a pump because they feel it may cause prospective partners to view their body or health status negatively.
- *Dependence on a mechanical device*: some people prefer not to depend on a mechanical device to maintain their health.
- *Trust/control*: it may take some time for pump users to trust their ability to manage their disease using a more complex treatment plan.

The potential psychological benefits of insulin pump use include those reported by individuals on injection-based intensive therapy: reduced anxiety and depres-sion, and improved quality of life (20). In addition, pump users with a history of poorly controlled diabetes report that the major advantage associated with pump treatment is a feeling of achievement in controlling their diabetes (21).

Individuals with visual and physical deficits may need assistance from friends and/or family, and those who live alone require more frequent SMBG to metic-ulously guard against severe and nocturnal hypoglycemia. One currently avail-able pump (MiniMed 506) has an alarm feature designed for those who live alone: the AUTO-OFF feature can be programmed to turn off the pump and sound an alarm if the person has not touched the pump within the programmed amount of time (which can vary from 1 to 18 hours). For example, if a pump user living alone were to become hypoglycemic and unable to manage the pump, it would stop delivering insulin automatically after the preset period of time.

Pump users with a history of poorly controlled diabetes report that the major advantage associated with pump treatment is a feeling of achievement in controlling their diabetes.

> "When my doctor prescribed an insulin pump, I thought it was going to be a ball and chain forever reminding me that I had this chronic disease. Instead, I discovered the pump was the key to my good health and allowed me, for the first time ever, to feel I was in control of my diabetes instead of feeling my diabetes controlled me."
>
> *Quote from a 35-year old woman after seven years of pump therapy*

FINANCIAL CONSIDERATIONS

The insulin pump is a more expensive insulin delivery system than multiple daily injections. Candidates for CSII need to have adequate financial resources in the form of health insurance or personal resources. Most health insurers will reimburse for the costs associated with insulin pump therapy if it can be documented that such treatment is medically necessary for the person. This often requires the individual to first attempt intensive control using a multiple daily injection regimen. If he or she fails to meet glycemic goals on MDI, then the third-party payor is more likely to approve reimbursement for the insulin pump.

CONTRAINDICATIONS TO INSULIN PUMP THERAPY

Certain behaviors are "red flags," signaling that someone may be a poor candidate for CSII (9):

- Lack of consistent blood glucose monitoring (less than four times per day)
- Unwillingness to calculate meal dosages
- Intense fear of needles or pain
- Extreme concern about hiding the pump from others
- Poor compliance with the treatment plan or scheduled visits
- Unwillingness to disclose diabetes to others
- Severe and unstable psychiatric conditions

While the above are not absolute contraindications, individuals exhibiting these behaviors should be carefully evaluated and encouraged to try a period of intensive treatment using multiple daily injections before attempting CSII. Individuals lacking the behavioral, mental, or physical ability to undertake an intensive diabetes management program or who have medical conditions that could be worsened with intensive control should not be considered for this form of therapy.

SUMMARY

Careful candidate selection is crucial to successful use of the insulin pump. Good candidates for CSII include those who are motivated to accept greater levels of responsibility for their own self-care, particularly those who have been unable to achieve adequate glycemic control or a more normal lifestyle with injection-based intensive management.

Pump therapy is best implemented with the support of a team of health care professionals who are trained in all aspects of diabetes management and CSII. The diabetologist, nurse educator, and dietitian are key team members; the social worker/ psychologist and exercise therapist are helpful adjuncts to the team. The most important member of the team is the pump user. With proper education, motivation, and support, the insulin pump user can safely achieve better blood glucose control and increased lifestyle flexibility.

REFERENCES

1. Teutsch SM, Herman WH, Dwyer DM, Lane JM. Mortality among diabetic patients using continuous subcutaneous insulin-infusion pumps. *N Engl J Med* 1984;310:361-368.

2. American Association of Diabetes Educators. Education for continuous subcutaneous insulin infusion pump users. *Diabetes Educ* 1986;13:10.

3. American Diabetes Association. Continuous subcutaneous insulin infusion. *Diabetes Care* 1993;16:2.

4. Schifferdecker E, Schmidt K, Boehm BO, Schatz H. Long-term compliance of intensified insulin therapy. *Diabetes Res Clin Pract* 1994;23:17-23.

5. Bode BW, Steed D, Davidson PC. Long-term pump use and SMBG in 205 patients. *Diabetes* 1994;43(Suppl 1):220A.

6. Marcus AO. Patient selection for insulin pump therapy. *Practical Diabetology* Nov 1992:12-18.

7. Strowig S. Initiation and management of insulin pump therapy. *Diabetes Educ* 1993;19:50-58.

8. Jennings AM, Lewis KS, Murdoch S, Talbot JF, Bradley C, Ward JD. Randomized trial comparing continuous subcutaneous insulin infusion and conventional insulin therapy in type II diabetic patients poorly controlled with sulfonylureas. *Diabetes Care* 1991;14:738-744.

9. Hirsch IB, Farkas-Hirsch R, Cryer PE. Continuous subcutaneous insulin infusion for the treatment of diabetic patients with hypoglycemia unawareness. *Diab Nutr Metab* 1991;4:41-43.

10. Farkas-Hirsch R, Hirsch IB. Continuous subcutaneous insulin infusion: a review of the past and its implementation for the future. *Diabetes Spectrum* 1994;7:80-84.

11. The DCCT Research Group. Effect of intensive treatment of diabetes on the development and progression of long-term complications in insulin- dependent diabetes mellitus. *N Engl J Med* 1993;329:977-986.

12. Kitzmiller JL, Gavin LA, Gin GD, Jovanovic-Peterson L, Main EK, Zigrang WD. Preconception care of diabetes glycemic control prevents congenital anomalies. *JAMA* 1991;265:731-736.

13. Kitzmiller J, Younger D, Hare J, Phillipe M, Vignati L,Fargnoli B, Grause A. Continuous subcutaneous insulin therapy during early pregnancy. *Obstet Gynecol* 1985;66:606-611.

14. Wredling R, Lins PE, Adamson U. Factors influencing the clinical outcome of continuous subcutaneous insulin infusion in routine practice. *Diabetes Res Clin Pract* 1993;19:59-67.

15. de Beaufort CE, Houtzager CMGJ, Bruining GJ, Aarsen RSR, Den Boer NC, Grose WFA, Van Strik R, De Visser JJ. Continuous subcutaneous insulin infusion (CSII) versus conventional injection therapy in newly diagnosed diabetic children: two-year followup of a randomized, prospective trial. *Diabet Med* 1989;6:766-771.

16. Slijper FME, de Beaufort CE, Bruining GJ, De Visser JJ, Aarsen RSR, Kicken DAM, Van Strik R. Psychological impact of continuous subcutaneous insulin infusion pump therapy in nonselected newly diagnosed insulin dependent (type I) diabetic children: evaluation after two years of therapy. *Diabete Metab* 1990;16:273-277.

17. Schiffrin A, Desrosiers M, Moffatt M, Belmonte MM. Feasibility of strict diabetes control in insulin-dependent diabetic adolescents. *J Pediatr* 1983;103:522-527.

18. Etkind ET. How to make pump therapy work. *Practical Diabetology* 1988;7:3-5.

19. Jornsay DL, Duckles AE, Hankinson JP. Psychological considerations for patient selection and adjustment to insulin pump therapy. *Diabetes Educ* 1988;14:291-296.

20. Mazze RS, Lucido D, Shamoon H. Psychological and social correlates of glycemic control. *Diabetes Care* 1984;7:360-366.

21. Foley-Nolan D, Foley-Nolan A, Temperley D, Devlin J. Diabetics treated with continuous subcutaneous insulin infusion pumps. *Ir Med J* 1989;82:159-160.

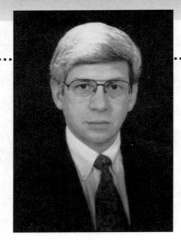

ROBERT J. TANENBERG, MD, FACP

Dr. Tanenberg is Clinical Associate Professor of Medicine at Georgetown University and Medical Director of the Diabetes Treatment Center at Washington Hospital Center in Washington, D.C. In his private endocrinology practice, he specializes in intensive management of patients with type I diabetes, in particular, adolescents, pregnant women, and adults with brittle diabetes. Dr. Tanenberg served as a consultant to the National Institutes of Health (NIH) for the Diabetes Control and Complications Trial. He has authored several articles and book chapters on diabetes management and lectures widely to both lay and professional audiences on diabetes treatment and insulin pump therapy. Since 1990, Dr. Tanenberg has been a principal investigator for the MiniMed Implantable Pump Program.

KAREN R. DAWN, RN, BSN, CDE

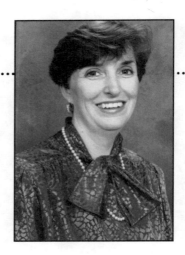

Ms. Dawn is a clinical nurse specialist and MiniMed certified insulin pump trainer with more than a decade of insulin pump experience. She works on the diabetes unit at Georgetown University Hospital, Washington, D.C., where she had previously served as Diabetes Research Nurse for many years. She also works as a diabetes nurse/educator in several Washington-area private practices, including that of Dr. Robert Tanenberg, and serves as coordinator for the MiniMed Implantable Pump study at the Washington Hospital Center in Washington, D.C. Ms. Dawn is a frequent lecturer on diabetes education and insulin pump therapy management. In 1994, she coauthored the Diabetes Patient Education Video Series with the American Association of Diabetes Educators.

INITIATING PUMP THERAPY

4

Beginning insulin pump therapy can be an exciting, yet anxious, time for the person with diabetes. Many aspects of the self-care routine will remain the same, but others will change. The new pump user will require reassurance, step-by-step education and continuing support from the diabetes care team, family and friends.

There are many different ways to initiate insulin pump therapy. We have included some guidelines that have assisted us over our years of initiating insulin pumps. The key to successful initiation of insulin pump therapy is an educated and motivated health care team. The team should consist of the physician, diabetes educator, registered dietitian and a counselor. All team members working together will help to make the transition from injection therapy to insulin pump therapy a smooth one.

INSULIN PUMP THERAPY CONTRACT

Because pump initiation is often a busy and hectic time for the pump user, it is very helpful to draw up an "Insulin Pump Therapy Contract," such as the one shown here, before initiating pump therapy. This agreement can be used to document that you have discussed the safety aspects of continuous subcutaneous insulin infusion (CSII) with the pump user and that he or she understands the specific self-care responsibilities that are required for successful pump use.

IN THIS CHAPTER

Pump Therapy Contract

Prepump Education

Inpatient and Outpatient Initiation

Infusion Site Care

INSULIN PUMP THERAPY CONTRACT

After consultation with my physician, I have chosen to use an insulin pump to help treat my diabetes. I understand the pump offers certain advantages to me in terms of normalization of lifestyle and improved control of my blood glucose levels, if used in accordance with my physician's instructions. I also understand improved control may help me to prevent the complications associated with diabetes. For these reasons and others, I have chosen the pump over other forms of treatment.

I understand I may be at higher risk for diabetic ketoacidosis when using an insulin pump. Although the pump has certain advantages, I recognize it is an electro-mechanical device that, like all other mechanical devices, may fail. It is still up to me to closely monitor my blood glucose levels to ensure that I am receiving the appropriate amount of insulin. In the event that my blood glucose levels rise and I am unable to normalize them with what seems an appropriate amount of insulin, I understand I must consult my health care team immediately. I recognize such an event may be caused by illness, stress, pump malfunction or other factors. Therefore, it is my responsibility to involve my health care team in helping me deal with unexplained high blood glucose levels as soon as possible.

I understand hypoglycemia is a risk with any form of diabetes therapy. I understand that symptoms of hypoglycemia are less apparent with better blood glucose control. I may be at increased risk for hypoglycemia if I do not check my blood glucose frequently, have increased activity, have decreased food intake, take too much bolus insulin, or drink alcohol. It is my responsibility to treat my hypoglycemia appropriately and to instruct my significant others in the storage and use of glucagon.

I have read and understand the following "Seven Ingredients for Successful Pumping."

Seven Ingredients for Successful Pumping

1. Enthusiastic physician
2. Informed diabetes educator
3. Pump user willing to take charge
4. Attention to detail by all involved
5. Minimum of four blood glucose tests per day
6. Rapid response to hypoglycemia (low blood glucose levels)
7. Rapid response to hyperglycemia (high blood glucose levels) by following these guidelines:
    a. Change infusion set if blood glucose is elevated two times in a row.
    b. Check ketones if blood glucose is above 250 mg/dL.
    c. Give an injection of insulin when nausea or vomiting occurs or if blood glucose remains elevated 2-3 hours after an infusion set change.
    d. Contact physician if vomiting occurs and/or if blood glucose remains elevated with ketones for 4 hours.

_____   _____

Pump User (Parent or Guardian)   Date   *Physician or Diabetes Educator   Date*

PREPUMP EDUCATION

Adequate prepump education is critical to successful initiation of pump therapy. Before beginning pump therapy, the person should receive comprehensive training in the principles of diabetes self-management and continuous subcutaneous insulin infusion. A significant other who learns all aspects of diabetes self-care and insulin pump therapy with the prospective pump user is a great asset.

The prospective pump user will benefit from having three preparatory visits with the diabetes educator (pump trainer) prior to initiating insulin pump therapy:

Visit One should include a review of the prospective pump user's diabetes history and a detailed overview of pump therapy. This visit typically lasts one to two hours. Discuss the advantages of CSII, realistic goals and expectations regarding pump therapy, and the precautions that must be taken when using a pump. Provide the prospective pump user with contact names and phone numbers for the dietitian, a counselor (if indicated), and other people using insulin pumps who may be able to help him or her finalize the decision to begin pump therapy.

Visit Two, scheduled after the individual receives the pump, focuses on detailed instruction in all aspects of pump use. Prior to the visit, encourage the pump user to read the pump instruction manual, watch the videotape, "play" with the buttons, and perform minor pump operations. The pump user needs to bring the pump to this visit, along with the pump *User's Guide,* two infusion sets, two reservoirs, the SportGuard™, dressing (if using the bent needle), alcohol swabs, and questions. (The pump trainer supplies the normal saline and Betadine.) Instruct the pump user in the operation of all pump programs, the filling of the reservoir with normal saline solution, the priming of the tubing, and insertion of the needle into the skin after cleansing it properly. Normal saline is used for at least three to four infusion set changes (six to twelve days) prior to insulin initiation.

Prior to pump initiation, the prospective pump user should also meet with a registered dietitian to obtain a personalized meal plan and learn how to count carbohydrates.

Visit Three is a follow-up visit at which the pump user's technique is reviewed, questions are answered, and knowledge is tested using the exam in the pump *User's Guide.* Insulin infusion is begun at this visit or within the next several days.

Prior to pump initiation, the prospective pump user should meet with a registered dietitian to obtain a personalized meal plan and learn how to count carbohydrates.

Prepump Training Topics

- Blood glucose target goals

- DKA prevention

- Hypoglycemia prevention

- Pump and infusion set operation

- Guidelines for basal rate and bolus adjustments

- Prevention of insertion site infection

- Handling sick days

- Everyday management

- Awareness of body image changes

Prepump Training Checklist

There are many elements involved in making a successful transition to pump therapy. Specific written guidelines for pump initiation can help document that critical tasks are completed. See the educational checklist at the back of this chapter for reference. This checklist should be signed by the diabetes educator and the pump user and placed in the chart.

Filling, Priming and Loading the Pump

Filling and priming the infusion set and pump are simple tasks; however, the pump user must practice them several times to develop proficiency. The MiniMed insulin pump syringe can be placed in the pump in one of two ways: the short-fill syringe method or the full-syringe method.

The short-fill method allows the syringe (reservoir) to be filled to 160 units and placed inside the pump so that the syringe neck is almost completely concealed within the pump case. Advantages of this method include:

- The smaller capacity serves as a reminder for timely infusion set changes.
- The smaller volume means insulin is exposed to body heat for a shorter time period, thus reducing the chance that it will lose potency.
- The luer neck is hidden inside the pump and, therefore, is less likely to "poke" the pump user when he or she bends over.

The short-fill method requires that a converter be placed in the pump as shown in the *User's Guide*. All MiniMed pumps are shipped from the factory in the short-fill mode.

The full-syringe method is for those individuals using more than 160 units of insulin within 48 hours. This method allows the syringe to be filled to its full capacity of 300 units.

PUMP INITIATION

CSII can be initiated safely and successfully in either an inpatient or an outpatient setting depending on the resources available and the needs of the pump user. Every pump user requires individualized support and ready access to the diabetes care team during pump initiation, regardless of the setting. The following conditions must be in place to ensure safe and effective pump initiation:

1. 24-hour access to the health care provider.

2. A friend or family member who is trained in diabetes care, glucagon administration, and pump use should be available to assist with the initiation.

3. Rigorous self-monitoring of blood glucose (premeal, bedtime, 12 AM, 3 AM and whenever symptoms of hyperglycemia or hypoglycemia occur).

4. Stable meal planning. Following a known, stable food pattern during the first weeks of pump use greatly simplifies the determination of basal rates and bolus doses.

5. Blood glucose meter calibration. A capillary finger-stick performed and read by the pump user should be compared to a blood glucose done by the laboratory in order to validate the user's technique and the instrument's accuracy. The glucose level measured in whole blood by the pump user is usually 15 percent lower than the laboratory measurement done on venous plasma.

Inpatient Initiation

Many inpatient diabetes units are equipped to provide the necessary training and supervision during CSII initiation. This includes making sure blood glucose determinations are performed at appropriate times, meal plans are reviewed by a registered dietitian, all insulin doses given by the pump are supervised, and all infusion set changes are monitored. With inpatient initiation, professional assistance is immediately available for handling any problems that may occur (1). Hospital stays may range from one to four days. Inpatient initiation is preferred, and often considered mandatory, for pregnant women, who require rapid normalization of glycemia as well as closely supervised initiation (2).

For inpatient pump starts, the following is a suggested protocol:

1. Determine time of admission. Admission can occur immediately prior to pump initiation if education and prepump training have been completed. Morning admission is generally preferable, as this allows full use of the first inpatient day.

2. Have patient's regular insulin for CSII ready and available prior to admission.

3. Obtain orders for the meal plan developed by the dietitian for the pump user. Discuss meal plan orders with the patient, the nurses and the dietary staff prior to admission. Food choices during the hospital stay must be as close to usual meals as possible for bolus adjustment to proceed appropriately. If necessary, write or obtain orders to specify "Do Not Change Patient Food Choices," or have patient choose foods from the hospital cafeteria.

4. Have patient limit exercise on the first several days of CSII initiation. This will allow for easier determination of the basal rate(s).

Confirm pump user's knowledge and skill regarding essential topics. Document instruction and learning assessment.

Outpatient initiation provides a more realistic setting for integrating pump routines into a person's lifestyle.

5. Start the pump using predetermined basal and bolus calculations (see Chapters 5, *Establishing & Verifying Basal Insulin Rates* and 6, *Bolus & Supplemental Insulin*).

6. Write or obtain specific orders for treatment of hypoglycemia.

7. Write or obtain orders to perform blood glucose testing before meals, at 10 PM, 12 AM, and 3 AM. These may be lab values or bedside glucose monitoring. The pump user should do parallel tests using his or her own meter to validate its accuracy.

8. Adjust basal rate in 0.1 U/h increments on the basis of the nighttime and prebreakfast readings (see Chapter 5, *Establishing & Verifying Basal Insulin Rates*).

9. Modify bolus doses on the basis of the next premeal blood glucose levels (see Chapter 6, *Bolus & Supplemental Insulin*).

10. Confirm the pump user's knowledge and skill regarding essential topics. Reinforce, correct and augment knowledge as needed. Document instruction and learning assessment.

11. Teach intramuscular injection technique for future reference.

12. Teach glucagon administration to a significant other.

13. Confirm postdischarge follow-up plan with the pump user before the end of the hospital stay.

Outpatient Initiation

Outpatient initiation provides a more realistic setting for integrating pump routines into a person's lifestyle. This mode of initiation is also preferred by some third-party reimbursement plans.

Outpatient insulin pump initiation protocols involve one to three days of office observation and teaching, coupled with intensive home monitoring and support. Morning pump starts are recommended in the outpatient setting to allow as much observation time in the office as possible before the new pump user returns home.

The following protocol may assist with initiating CSII in the outpatient setting:

1. Thoroughly review with the pump user all aspects of CSII troubleshooting.

2. Closely observe the pump user's ability to set up the pump for insulin initiation.

3. Have the person obtain his or her regular insulin for CSII prior to initiation.

4. Start the insulin pump, using predetermined basal and bolus calculations (see Chapters 5, *Establishing & Verifying Basal Insulin Rates* and 6, *Bolus & Supplemental Insulin*).

5. Check blood glucose every two hours during the day, with the pump user remaining in the office for observation. Provide written instructions detailing additional tests to be done after returning home. Recommended testing times include before meals, at bedtime, and at 12 AM and 3 AM (before returning to the office for the second day of the initiation program).

6. Arrange for the pump user to have 24-hour access to a member of the pump team. Provide specific instructions regarding when and how the pump user can reach a health care team member in the event that blood glucose readings fall outside the set parameters.

7. Have the pump user limit exercise for the first several days of CSII initiation. This will allow for easier determination of basal rate(s).

8. Include the spouse or significant other in these discussions.

9. Notify the on-call physician of the new pump user's status.

10. While the pump user is in the office, confirm his or her knowledge and skill regarding essential topics. Reinforce, correct and augment knowledge as needed. Document instruction and learning assessment.

11. Adjust basal rate in 0.1 U/h increments on the basis of the 12 AM, 3 AM, and prebreakfast blood glucose readings.

12. After the basal rate is confirmed, modify bolus doses on the basis of the next premeal blood glucose levels.

13. Confirm that the pump user has a Glucagon Emergency Kit and that the spouse or significant other who will be present during the initiation period knows how and when to use it.

14. Teach intramuscular injection technique for future reference.

WEANING FROM LONG- AND INTERMEDIATE-ACTING INSULIN

With either inpatient or outpatient initiation, "weaning" from conventional insulin is necessary. Modified insulin may take several days to clear from the system. Therefore, Ultralente insulin should be discontinued at least 24 hours prior to pump initiation, and NPH and Lente insulins should be discontinued 18 to 20 hours prior to initiation of pump therapy. Each new pump user's transition from conventional injections to CSII will need to be closely monitored.

NPH and Lente insulins should be discontinued 18 to 20 hours prior to initiation of pump therapy

During the lapse between conventional insulin administration and pump initiation, regular insulin should be injected every six hours to supply basal, bolus and corrective supplemental doses. This regular insulin could be given before meals, at midnight with a snack, and again at 6 AM. On the morning of pump initiation, to prevent an overlap between injected and infused insulins, the individual should take a prebreakfast injection of 10 to 20 percent less than the normal dose and NO NPH or Lente insulin. This will reduce the risk of hypoglycemia during initiation.

Every effort should be made to avoid hypoglycemia when a person is just beginning pump therapy. Careful insulin management with frequent blood glucose monitoring can help avoid a hypoglycemic episode that might shake a pump user's confidence during this vulnerable period. Blood glucose goals for the initial days of CSII should be in the upper normal ranges, as many pump users are less physically active than usual during their first few days of CSII.

INFUSION SITE CARE

Site Selection and Rotation

Proper infusion site selection and rotation promote predictable insulin absorption, protect infusion sites from undesirable tissue changes, and help prevent infection. The abdomen is the preferred area for placement of the infusion set, as insulin absorption from this area is faster, more predictable, and less affected by exercise than it is from other body areas. The upper outer thighs and hips also work reasonably well, as does the arm, although many people find dealing with the needle and tubing quite awkward with an arm placement. When these sites are used, care must be exercised to assure that needle placement is subcutaneous, not intramuscular, and frequent site inspections must be made to check for dislodgement due to these areas having more shear with clothing.

The more sites used, the less often any one site is injected, and the better assurance the pump user will have of keeping tissue healthy over the years. Therefore, no matter which body area is used–abdomen, thigh, hip or arm–the exact site within the area should be changed each time the infusion set is changed. The new site should be at least one inch away from the previous site, yet still convenient for needle/cannula placement. Areas to be avoided include: around the belt or waistline, at bikini/underwear lines, within a one-inch circle around the umbilicus, and any area where clothing would rub or constrict.

Infusion Site Preparation

To help prevent skin infections, the infusion site should be cleansed carefully and allowed to dry before inserting the bent needle or Sof-set™ and applying the tape.

Instruct the pump user to prepare the infusion site as follows:

1. Wash hands with soap and water.

The more sites used, the less often any one site is injected, and the better assurance the pump user will have of keeping tissue healthy over the years.

2. Avoid touching the tip of the reservoir (pump syringe), the end of the infusion set, or the top of the insulin bottle. Avoid breathing, blowing, or fanning directly over the pump, reservoir, infusion set, or site.

3. Scrub the infusion site with an antiseptic solution. Suggested solutions are chlorohexidine (Hibiclens), 1 to 2 percent iodine (Betadine Solution), or 90 percent alcohol. Cleanse skin in a circular fashion moving from inside the circle outward. The site cleansed should be the size of a tennis ball. Allow the site to air-dry. (If any localized skin irritation occurs, switching cleansing products may eliminate the problem.)

4. Insert infusion set (straight needle, bent needle or Sof-set) according to directions.

5. Apply a sterile dressing such as Polyskin (available from MiniMed Technologies), Tegaderm, Bio-occlusive, or Opsite securely to protect the site.

6. Change the infusion site every 48 hours. Change the set and site immediately if blood glucose readings are over 240 mg/dL twice in a row. (Individualize for pump user and circumstances.)

7. Check the infusion site with each void for dislodgement, redness, swelling, or bleeding. If these or other symptoms occur at the site, change the infusion set and site immediately.

8. If inflammation occurs, change the infusion site. This site should not be used again until the inflammation and swelling have cleared. Call your diabetes care team if the inflamed site is larger than a dime.

Skin Infections

Skin infections are a potential, but preventable, risk of pump therapy. In the Mason Clinic report, infection occurred at a frequency of one event per 27 patient months (3). More than half of the individuals with one skin infection had a second episode, and most infections appeared as cellulitis rather than abscesses. In the few abscesses that appeared, cultures revealed *Staphylococcus aureus* bacteria. Those individuals with infected infusion sites were more likely to be nasal carriers of S. *aureus* than were pump users without infected sites.

If a pump user is having recurrent site infections, he or she should be observed cleansing the site and changing the infusion set. If the cleansing and insertion techniques are acceptable, the pump user should add a topical antiseptic to the site preparation routine. If infusion site infections are still a problem in spite of careful cleansing and use of an antiseptic, the problem may be caused by S. *aureus*. If a nasal culture for S. *aureus* is positive, antibiotic may be applied topically to the nostrils or taken orally to help prevent or control infections.

In the case of active infection, the reservoir and infusion set must be removed and discarded and another infusion site used until the infection has cleared. Treatment with oral antibiotics is indicated, and application of warm, moist heat to the affected area for 20 minutes, four times per day, can accelerate healing. Use of a topical antibiotic cream early in the course of an infection will often slow or prevent its spread.

SELECTION AND USE OF INFUSION SET

Personal preference plays a key role in the choice of either Sof-set or Polyfin bent needle as the infusion set. If the pump user chooses the Sof-set, he or she should also have a straight or bent needle on hand and know when and how to use it.

The Sof-set

The Sof-set is similar to the intravenous angiocatheter in its insertion. It is a flexible teflon cannula which uses a metal needle to guide it into the subcutaneous tissue. After proper insertion and application to the skin, the introducer needle is removed and the flexible teflon cannula stays in place.

Advantages of the Sof-set include greater comfort, less irritation, and less risk of bleeding at the infusion site and into the tubing.

Advantages of the Sof-set include greater comfort, less irritation, and less risk of bleeding at the infusion site and into the tubing (which could occlude the tubing). Some pump users are able to leave the Sof-set in longer than a metal needle because it causes less local irritation and comes with an antibacterial dressing that may prevent an infection.

Proper Sof-set insertion technique is vital. Encourage the individual to review the instructions in the package insert. The following tips will help pump users avoid some common problems:

1. Before removing the Sof-set introducer needle, the pump user should give it a slight turn. This helps ensure that the cannula stays in place as the introducer needle is taken out.

2. Crimping is usually the result of improper insertion. If the pump user follows Method 1 described in the Sof-set package insert, the set MUST be inserted in a quick motion. By keeping the index finger on the needle hub during insertion, the pump user can apply sufficient pressure as the needle is pushed in. Pinching up the skin helps to stabilize it for quick, smooth insertion. If a pump user has problems inserting the needle quickly, he or she can try Method 2 described in the package insert.

3. Cannula bends can be caused by either improper insertion or loosening of the tape due to poor adhesion. The Sof-set can be stabilized by using a second piece of tape to cover the needle hub. This is particularly useful during exercise and sports when perspiration may reduce tape's sticking properties. Resistance from muscle tissue can also cause an "L" shaped bend in the cannula.

Metal Needle

A major advantage of using bent or straight metal needles is that pump users are more aware of their placement. With rigid needles, there is less chance of improper placement, as an incorrectly inserted or dislodged needle will cause discomfort. Metal needles may be more suitable for very thin people and in areas of the body with very little subcutaneous tissue.

Users of metal needles may experience soreness or irritation at the insertion site due to the rigidity of the needle or sensitivity to the metal.

Quick Release™ Infusion Connector

The Quick Release infusion connector is a relatively new option that allows simple disconnection from the pump. This can be particularly useful during showering, swimming, shopping and trying on clothes, sexual activity, or during periods when pump removal is required, such as during a CAT scan or MRI. See Chapter 9, *Everyday Management* for more information on the Quick Release.

Discomfort During Insertion

A small number of people experience discomfort when first inserting the infusion set. Some nurses recommend rubbing the area with ice to numb it slightly before inserting the needle. Another recommendation is to use a product called Emla Cream, a topical analgesic (pain killer) available from Astra USA, (800-228-EMLA). The cream is applied one hour before, and is washed off just before inserting the infusion set. The site should be clean and dry before insertion as previously described. Complete instructions for use are provided in the package insert for Emla Cream.

When to Change the Infusion Set

The infusion set and site should be changed frequently and regularly. A general rule of thumb is that a metal needle should be changed every two days, while a Sof-set should be changed at least every three days. The infusion set and site should also be changed whenever there is any irritation or discomfort at the infusion site or whenever two unexplained high blood glucose readings occur in a row. Leaving the set in for too long may promote hypertrophy (hardening of the skin tissue), leading to poor absorption of insulin, and will also increase the risk of infection.

The Quick Release™ infusion connector is a relatively new option that allows simple disconnection from the pump.

The best time to change an infusion set is right before giving a premeal bolus. This way, the bolus of insulin will clear away any tissue from the cannula or needle. The blood glucose level should be checked two to three hours after insertion. Advise the pump user not to change the infusion set at bedtime, as he or she will need to be awake for several hours after insertion to assess for proper insulin delivery.

SUMMARY

Successful initiation of pump therapy requires that the new pump user receive thorough prepump training in intensive diabetes management and all aspects of insulin pump therapy, and that the diabetes care team follow a comprehensive and systematic inpatient or outpatient initiation protocol. Use of an Insulin Pump Therapy Contract is encouraged prior to pump initiation to document that the pump user understands the potential risks of pump therapy and has been informed of his or her responsibilities, as well as those of the provider. Elements of successful pump therapy, covered throughout this book, need to be communicated in detail during pump initiation. This chapter places particular emphasis on proper infusion site care, which can help the pump user achieve consistent insulin absorption and avoid skin infection.

REFERENCES

1. American Association of Diabetes Educators. Position statement: education for continuous subcutaneous insulin infusion pump users. *Diabetes Educ* 1986;13:10.

2. Farkas-Hirsch R, Hirsch IB. Continuous subcutaneous insulin infusion: a review of the past and its implementation for the future. *Diabetes Spectrum* 1994;7:80-84.

3. Mecklenburg RS, Benson EA, Benson JW, Fredlund PN, Guinn T, Metz RJ, Nielsen RL, Sannar CA. Acute complications associated with insulin infusion pump therapy. Report of experience with 161 patients. *JAMA* 1984;252:3265-3269.

EDUCATIONAL CHECKLIST FOR CSII INITIATION

	Instructed Date/Initial Comments	Successfully Completed Date/Initial Comments
Prepump Education:		
1. State advantages of CSII		
2. State change in body image		
3. List ways to overcome body image changes		
4. Explain increased risk of diabetic ketoacidosis		
5. Describe the potential change in hypoglycemic awareness		
Pump Operation:		
1. Watch pump video		
2. Read instruction manual; identify troubleshooting page		
3. Change batteries		
4. Basic programming		
a. Select button function		
b. Activate button function		
c. Use of up and down arrows		
5. Set time and day of the week		
6. Bolus		
a. Check last 7 meal boluses		
b. Set meal bolus		
c. Stop meal bolus during delivery		
7. Suspend mode (use & beep notification)		
8. Basal rate(s)		
a. Review current rate		
b. Review number of profiles		
c. Review setting profiles		
d. How to cancel profiles		
9. Temporary rate		
a. When to use		
b. Notification of its use		
c. How to cancel		
10. Daily totals (last 7 days)		
11. Set-up options		
a. Maximum bolus (factory 10.0 U)		
b. Maximum basal rate (factory 2.0 U/h)		
c. Time display format (factory AM/PM)		
d. Insulin concentration (factory U-100) *Note–this change clears all memory*		
e. Automatic off safety setting (factory = off). Useful safety mechanism for pump users living alone.		

	Instructed Date/Initial Comments	Successfully Completed Date/Initial Comments

Preparing Insulin Infusion:

1. Fill the syringe
2. Prime infusion set
3. Check for air bubbles
4. Syringe placement
   a. Know short vs full syringe method
   b. Use 5.0 unit bolus to take up the "slack"
5. Needle insertion
   a. Identify possible sites
   b. Prep site with ____
   c. Insert needle (Sof-set or metal)
   d. Apply sterile dressing ____
   e. Give 0.5 unit bolus to clear the needle/cannula after insertion
   f. Turn needle and remove from Sof-set

Troubleshooting:

1. Alarms
   a. Review alarm card
   b. Understand difference between Alarm & Error messages
   c. A-35 (motion sensor alarm)
   d. Overinfusion alarm (review maximums)
2. High blood glucose levels
   a. Review possible causes: Loss of insulin potency, bolus too small, site used too long, improper timing of bolus, illness, leaks or air in tubing, crimps in the cannula, poor absorption from site.
   b. Change infusion set if high blood glucoses occur twice in a row
   c. Give insulin by regular syringe SQ
   d. Check for ketones and call physician
3. Low blood glucose - treat first
   a. Review possible causes: Infrequent blood glucose measurements, bolus too large, low carbohydrate meal, increased exercise.
   b. Preventive techniques: Check glucose often, especially before a meal and before driving a car; always carry quick-acting carbohydrates
   c. Review glucagon administration with family members

Daily Use Instructions:

1. Infusion sets
   a. Change set every ____ days
   b. Preventive site examinations

	Instructed Date/Initial Comments	Successfully Completed Date/Initial Comments
2. Showering, bathing, swimming & sports		
a. Quick Release		
b. SportGuard & other examples		
3. Blood glucose monitoring		
a. Check a minimum of 4 times per day		
b. Know when to increase monitoring times		
c. ALWAYS check before bed!		
4. Bolus times before meals		
a. If glucose is normal ____		
b. If glucose is high ____		
c. If glucose is low ____		
d. At restaurants, etc. ____		
5. Bolus algorithms		
a. How much extra to take for a high glucose		
b. How much extra/less to take when varying meal size		
c. How much less to take for a low blood glucose		
6. Wearing the pump		
a. Use of belt clip & leather case		
b. Other concealment options		
7. Sick days		
a. Monitor blood glucose every 2 hours		
b. Give written protocols		
c. Know when to call physician		
8. Switch to conventional delivery		
a. Record on a card doses needed if pump becomes inoperable		
9. 24-hour hotline		
a. Phone number on back of pump		
b. MiniMed business hours are 8AM - 5PM Pacific Standard Time; Clinical Services Rep. will be paged for all after-hours emergencies		
c. When to call MiniMed vs when to call physician		
10. Supplies		
a. List of supplies needed		
b. Know where to order supplies		
c. List items you "must have with you at all times"		

_____   _____

Pump User Signature   *Date*   *Diabetes Educator*   *Date*

CHAPTER AUTHOR

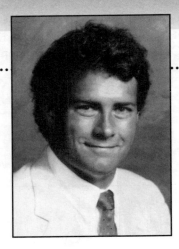

BRUCE W. BODE, MD

An internationally known speaker and author on insulin pump therapy, Dr. Bode is in private practice with the Atlanta Diabetes Associates and serves as Medical Director, Diabetes Treatment Center at West Paces Medical Center, Atlanta, GA. He also serves as President of the American Diabetes Association, Georgia Affiliate, and is on the Board of Directors for the Juvenile Diabetes Foundation, Atlanta chapter.

ESTABLISHING & VERIFYING BASAL RATES 5

In a healthy, non-diabetic person, the pancreas produces the correct amount of insulin to maintain homeostasis. This basal, or background, insulin regulates the production and availability of fats, carbohydrates and proteins under fasting conditions, and accounts for between 40 and 50 percent of the body's total daily insulin requirement. When carbohydrates are taken by a person with a normal pancreas, insulin is released into the bloodstream rapidly and at a level that precisely matches the carbohydrate content of the meal. This insulin release, called a bolus, comprises the balance of the total daily insulin need.

The person with optimally controlled type I diabetes must provide the correct amount of insulin to cover these needs, either by multiple daily injections (MDI) or the use of an insulin pump. An insulin pump, when compared to MDI, offers the advantage of covering basal and bolus needs separately.

An insulin pump provides the most precise way to mimic normal basal insulin secretion by delivering small amounts of regular insulin on a continuous basis. If necessary, alternate rates can be programmed to accommodate individual basal rate requirements, making optimal glycemic control easier.

ESTABLISHING THE INITIAL BASAL INSULIN DOSE

Pump therapy is initiated using a single basal rate, although approximately 60 percent of pump users may require the addition of a second basal rate to cover increased insulin requirements

IN THIS CHAPTER

Calculating Initial Rate

Testing the Overnight Rate

Evaluating Daytime & Evening Rates

Basal Rate Tips

during the dawn hours (1). The initial basal rate can be determined using either the total prepump insulin dose or the person's body weight.

Calculation Based on the Total Prepump Insulin Dose

In our practice we have found that most pump users require approximately 25 percent less insulin than their total prepump insulin dose at pump initiation and, long-term, stabilize at a 15 to 17 percent reduction relative to the total daily prepump dose (unpublished data 1994). Calculation of the initial basal insulin dose, therefore, begins with reducing the total daily prepump dose by 25 percent. For example, the initial total pump insulin dose for a person whose prepump total was 40 units would be 30 units.

Basal insulin comprises approximately 50 percent of this new dose, with boluses accounting for the remainder. In the previous example, the basal insulin would be 15 units, and this value would be divided by 24 hours to yield an initial basal rate of 0.6 unit per hour, as follows:

Total prepump insulin dose	= 40 U
Reduce total daily dose by 25% (40 x 75%)	= 30 U
Basal insulin dose (30 U x 50%)	= 15 U
Hourly basal rate (15 U/24 h)	= 0.6 U/h

Some persons may require a slightly lower percentage of their daily insulin in the form of basal. Preadolescent children, for example, tend to have a higher caloric intake, which needs to be matched with larger insulin boluses. Therefore, they may require only 40 percent of their daily insulin in the form of basal and 60 percent in the form of boluses.

Calculation Based on Current Body Weight

If there is concern that the person's prepump total daily insulin dose is incorrect, as evidenced by persistent hypo- or hyperglycemia, the starting basal rate should also be estimated on the basis of current body weight. A safe starting dose for the basal rate can be calculated by using 0.22 unit per kilogram per day (or 0.1 unit per pound per day). This formula provides a basal rate at the lower end of normal, which can then be adjusted upwards as needed.

If the estimated basal rate based on the prepump dose does not agree with that based on body weight, the LOWER rate should be chosen for initiation.

VERIFYING THE BASAL RATE

The basal rate is set correctly if blood glucose levels remain in the target range under fasting conditions, defined as no food or bolus insulin for at least five hours. Target blood glucose ranges should be individually established based on the person's history of severe hypoglycemia, the presence of reduced hypoglycemia awareness, and other pertinent factors (2). Guideline target blood glucose ranges are listed in the accompanying table.

Calculation of the initial basal insulin dose begins with reducing the total daily prepump dose by 25 percent.

GUIDELINE TARGET BLOOD GLUCOSE RANGES (mg/dL)

Clinical History	Premeal	Bedtime
No hypoglycemia	70-150	80-150
Reduced hypoglycemia aware-ness or cardiovascular disease	80-160	100-160
Recurrent severe hypoglycemia	100-200	120-200

VERIFYING THE OVERNIGHT BASAL RATE

Verifying overnight blood glucose levels provides an early indication of the appropriateness of the initial single basal rate. It also permits early recognition of any nocturnal hypoglycemia or increased dawn insulin need that would necessitate prompt adjustment of the basal profile.

To verify the overnight basal rate, the pump user should eat three meals of equal carbohydrate content and eliminate the bedtime snack. The overnight period is broken into three test "windows," as follows:

Bedtime: 9 PM - midnight
Night: Midnight - 3 AM
Dawn: 3 AM - 7 AM

(These windows are for a person who eats at 7 AM, 12 noon, and 5 PM and sleeps from 10 PM to 6 AM. Times should be adjusted for other schedules.) Blood glucose is checked at 9 PM, midnight, 3 AM, and 7 AM. If the blood glucose level changes by 30 mg/dL or more in any window, the basal rate for that window is adjusted up or down by 0.1 unit per hour two to three hours prior to that blood glucose change (3).

For example:
- If the blood glucose at midnight is 100 mg/dL and at 3 AM is 70 mg/dL, the basal rate is decreased by 0.1 unit per hour beginning at midnight or 1 AM.
- If the blood glucose at midnight is 100 mg/dL and at 3 AM is 140 mg/dL, the basal rate is increased by 0.1 unit per hour starting at midnight or 1 AM.

An exception occurs if there is a significant dawn rise (from 3 AM to 7 AM) the first night of pump initiation. If such a rise occurs, a second basal rate (Profile 2), equal to two times the initial basal rate, should be initiated at 3 AM or 4 AM for a period of six hours to cover the dawn rise. Following this six-hour period (at about 9 AM or 10 AM), the basal rate should be reset (Profile 3) to the primary rate. An example 24-hour basal insulin profile in a person with the dawn phenomenon might be as follows:

Basal Profile	Basal Rate	Time Period
1	0.6 U/h	Midnight - 3 AM
2	1.2 U/h	3 AM - 9 AM
3	0.6 U/h	9 AM - Midnight

To verify the accuracy of the dawn basal rate, the pump user should test the blood glucose at midnight and 3 AM every other night for the first week following initiation of the dawn basal. If the blood glucose changes by more than 30 mg/dL, the dawn basal rate should be increased or decreased accordingly by 0.1 unit per hour.

Approximately two weeks after starting CSII, the pump user should evaluate both the rate and duration of the dawn basal insulin. This requires skipping the breakfast meal and the prebreakfast bolus and testing the blood glucose every two hours during the morning "window," from 7 AM until noon. If there is an increase or decrease of 30 mg/dL or more in blood glucose during this period, adjustment of the basal rate, or its duration, is indicated. Guidelines are as follows:

- If the 7 AM blood glucose is in the target range, but the 9 AM blood glucose is low by more than 30 mg/dL, the dawn basal rate needs to be ended earlier: end the dawn basal rate (Profile 2) and begin the morning basal rate (Profile 3) at 7 AM.

- If the blood glucose rises from 7 AM until 9 AM, the basal rate during this period should be increased. End the dawn basal rate (Profile 2) at 7 AM and begin a new basal rate, Profile 3, which should be equal to the dawn basal rate plus 0.1 unit per hour. End Profile 3 at 9 AM and revert back to the original rate (Profile 4). To illustrate:

Basal Profile	Basal Rate	Time Period
1	0.6 U/h	Midnight - 3 AM
2	1.2 U/h	3 AM - 7 AM
3	1.3 U/h	7 AM - 9 AM
4	0.6 U/h	9 AM - Midnight

- If the dawn basal rate (Profile 2) ends at 9 AM and the blood glucose is high by 30 mg/dL or more at 11 AM, one could either extend the duration of the dawn basal (Profile 2) by one hour or increase the morning rate (Profile 3) by 0.1 unit per hour.

EVALUATING THE DAYTIME AND EVENING BASAL RATE

There is seldom any need to test the basal rate through the balance of the day. However, unexplained high or low blood glucose readings in the afternoon or evening hours may indicate a need to test additional "windows" as follows:

- *Afternoon: Noon - Supper (5 PM)*
  The pump user should take the prebreakfast bolus and eat breakfast before 7 AM. Lunch and its bolus are skipped. The blood glucose is tested at noon, 2 PM, and 5 PM. If the blood glucose changes by more than 30 mg/dL, the pump user should make a corresponding 0.1 unit per hour adjustment in the basal rate beginning two hours before the change in blood glucose.

- *Evening: Supper (5 PM) - Bedtime (10 PM)*
  The pump user should take the prelunch bolus and eat lunch before noon. Dinner and its bolus are skipped. The blood glucose is tested at 5 PM, 7 PM, and 10 PM. If the blood glucose changes by more than 30 mg/dL, the pump user should make a corresponding 0.1 unit per hour adjustment in the basal rate beginning two hours before the change in blood glucose.

REASSESSING BASAL RATES

Once established, basal rates seldom need to be changed. Adjusting basal rates frequently in response to elevated blood glucose levels, especially during the day, complicates insulin dynamics and can make it difficult to analyze patterns and make appropriate adjustments. The majority of pump users (>95 percent) achieve good glycemic control with three or fewer basal rates per day (unpublished data, 1994).

Basal rates should, however, be reevaluated when any of the following occurs:

1. **Significant, sustained change in activity**
   Increased activity decreases the insulin requirement; conversely, decreased activity is likely to raise the basal insulin requirement. For example, if the pump user changes from an active occupation to one less active, or vice-versa, basal insulin may require adjustment. If the change in activity is temporary (i.e., several hours), a temporary basal rate can be used. Refer to Chapter 10, *Exercise and the Pump*, for details on the use of temporary basal rates.

2. **Significant change in weight**
   A gain or loss of 5 to 10 percent or more of body weight may change the basal insulin requirement. Upon starting a weight-loss diet, a reduction in the basal rate of 10 to 30 percent will be required.

The majority of pump users (>95 percent) achieve good glycemic control with three or fewer basal rates per day.

A temporary basal rate increase can be used during illness to meet extreme insulin requirements.

3. **Gastroparesis**

   Damage to the nerves controlling the peristalsis of the intestines causes food to be absorbed more slowly. This delay commonly causes problems in glycemic control. When a person with gastroparesis takes a premeal bolus, hypoglycemia can occur two to three hours later, followed by hyperglycemia. In this situation, use of a higher temporary basal rate for three hours after the meal, rather than a premeal bolus, may be helpful (4). Alternatively, the bolus might be taken after the meal.

4. **Pregnancy**

   Insulin requirements change constantly as pregnancy progresses. The need to strictly avoid nocturnal hypoglycemia and morning ketosis may require a lower nighttime basal rate from midnight to 3 AM, followed by an increase of two to three times that level in the dawn hours. During the second and third trimesters of pregnancy, basal and bolus doses may need to be changed every few days as determined by blood glucose measurements. For more detailed information regarding pregnancy and pumps, refer to Chapter 13, *Pump Therapy in Preconception and Pregnancy*.

BASAL RATE TIPS

- The ideal basal rate is one that keeps the fasting* blood glucose level within the target range. If the basal rate requires adjustment, the change should be initiated two hours BEFORE the blood glucose begins to rise or fall.

- Multiple basal rates may be necessary

- Indications that the basal rate is too HIGH include:
  - Any low blood glucose level during the night or before breakfast.
  - Unexplained lows during the day when a meal is delayed or skipped.

- Indications that the basal rate is too LOW include:
  - Elevated fasting or 3 AM blood glucose values with normal bedtime blood glucose value.
  - Increased blood glucose when a meal is skipped or delayed.

- Periodically, the total basal and bolus doses should be checked to ensure that neither is greater than 60 percent of the total daily dose of insulin.

Fasting is defined as no food or bolus insulin for 5 hours.

---

5. **Menses**

   Blood glucose levels can rise substantially in the days preceding menstruation and then drop again or vary throughout menses (5). Women should carefully assess blood glucose profiles surrounding the menses, adjusting the basal dose(s) as needed.

6. **Illness**

   Higher basal rates are often needed to combat the added stress produced by illness or infection. For example, bacterial infections may cause the total daily insulin requirement to double. Blood glucose levels during short-term viral illnesses are more easily controlled by using supplemental boluses, rather than by raising the basal rate(s). However, a temporary basal rate increase can be used during illness to meet extreme insulin requirements. With resolution of the illness, the person should reduce basal or bolus doses to customary levels to avoid an insulin reaction.

7. **Medications**

   Drugs such as prednisone are known to increase blood glucose levels and, therefore, to increase the need for insulin. The pump user should make sure that the physician prescribing the drug(s) is aware of his or her diabetes, and must also notify the diabetes team so they will recommend proper insulin adjustments.

8. **Exercise**

   Although people respond differently to exercise, the more strenuous and/or prolonged the exercise, the more likely that a drop in blood glucose will occur. This drop in blood glucose can be balanced with a temporary lowering of the basal rate or by reducing premeal boluses. Temporary basal insulin reductions are ideal for moderate or strenuous exercise lasting 60 minutes or more, and are also helpful in preventing postexercise hypoglycemia. For more information regarding exercise and the use of pumps, see Chapter 10, *Exercise and the Pump*.

Establishing and verifying an accurate basal insulin profile is essential to maintaining target blood glucose levels.

SUMMARY

Establishing and verifying an accurate basal insulin profile is essential to maintaining target blood glucose levels. Multiple basal rates may be necessary for optimal, 24–hour glycemic control. When verifying the initial basal rate profile, it is recommended to begin with the overnight period. This both eliminates the need to skip meals and permits early recognition of any increased dawn insulin need or nocturnal hypoglycemia. Daytime and evening basal rates seldom need to be changed, but may require adjustment under certain conditions. The insulin pump allows convenient and precise modification of the basal profile to meet the individual needs of the pump user.

REFERENCES

1. Bode B, Steed D, Davidson P. Long-term pump use and SMBG in 205 patients. *Diabetes* 1994;43(Suppl 1):220A.

2. Hirsch IB, Farkas-Hirsch R. Skyler JS. Intensive insulin therapy for treatment of type I diabetes. *Diabetes Care* 1990;13:1265-1283.

3. Hildebrandt P, Birch K, Jensen BM, Kuhl C. Subcutaneous insulin infusion: change in basal infusion rate has no immediate effect on insulin absorption rate. *Diabetes Care* 1986;9:561-564.

4. Barnett JL, Vinik AI. Gastrointestinal disturbances. In: Lebovitz HE, ed. *Therapy for Diabetes Mellitus and Related Disorders*, Second Edition. Alexandria, VA: American Diabetes Association; 1994:289-292.

5. Moberg E, Kollind M., Lins P-E, Adamson U. Day-to-day variation of insulin sensitivity in patients with type 1 diabetes: role of gender and menstrual cycle. *Diabet Med* 1995;12:224-228.

CHAPTER AUTHOR

6

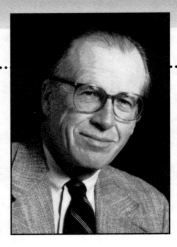

PAUL C. DAVIDSON, MD, CDE

Dr. Davidson is Medical Director of the Diabetes Treatment Center of America at West Paces Ferry Hospital, Atlanta, Georgia, and serves on the DTCA's Medical Advisory Council. He is also a founding partner and private practitioner in Atlanta Diabetes Associates, Atlanta, GA, an endocrinology group practice providing primary and consultative care for persons with diabetes. Dr. Davidson served as Associate Editor of *Annals of Internal Medicine* from 1976 to 1978. A developer of the Glucommander insulin infusion program, Dr. Davidson became a principal investigator for the MiniMed Implantable Pump Program in 1990. He firmly believes in the use of the insulin pump for controlling diabetes – to date, his center has placed over 600 patients on the pump.

BOLUS & SUPPLEMENTAL INSULIN

6

Insulin is rapidly released from the pancreas into the bloodstream when food is eaten by a non-diabetic individual. This **bolus** insulin has a separate and distinct function from the basal insulin necessary for maintaining homeostasis. Bolus insulin is related to the "glycemic effect" (the effect on blood glucose) of the food(s) eaten, and thus maintains normoglycemia. As most of the glycemic effect of food is due to carbohydrate, the bolus insulin released by the pancreas (the islet cell response) is largely determined by the carbohydrate content of the meal.

Premeal bolus insulin delivery by a pump mimics the normal islet cell response. That is, the amount of carbohydrate eaten in a meal relates to the amount of insulin needed. There is, however, one major difference: insulin delivered by continuous subcutaneous insulin infusion (CSII) does not enter the bloodstream directly. It is administered into the subcutaneous tissue. This delays the insulin's effect on blood glucose levels, and makes the timing of bolus insulin delivery an important factor in successful glycemic control (1-3).

Using an insulin pump allows greater flexibility in meal timing. If the pump user decides to skip a meal, the bolus is omitted. If a meal is larger or smaller than usual, a larger or smaller insulin bolus is given (4-6). The pump also offers the benefit of delivering insulin in fractions of a unit. This increased precision permits careful matching of bolus doses to insulin need and reduces the risk of overinsulinization.

IN THIS CHAPTER

Initial Bolus Dose

Timing of Boluses

Supplemental Doses

Calculating the Sensitivity Factor with the "1500" Rule

Supplemental bolus insulin (supplement) is a term commonly used to describe the insulin given to lower occasional high blood glucose levels when they occur, or to adjust premeal boluses if the individual's blood glucose level is below his or her target range. A supplemental insulin dose can be estimated from a formula based on the person's target blood glucose levels and his or her sensitivity to insulin.

PREMEAL BOLUSES

Setting the Initial Bolus Dose

At pump initiation, 40 to 50 percent of the total daily insulin dose is given as a single basal rate (See Chapter 5, *Establishing & Verifying Basal Rates*), with the remaining 50 to 60 percent given as premeal boluses. Initially dividing the premeal insulin into three equal boluses for three meals of equal carbohydrate content, with no bedtime snack, allows for a more effective analysis of the insulin requirement. Following a known, stable food pattern during the first few weeks of pump use is necessary to adjust basal rates. A stable meal plan also allows for the estimation of an accurate carbohydrate to insulin ratio for determining appropriate premeal boluses.

A sample calculation of the initial bolus dose is found in Table 1.

Table 1

EXAMPLE CALCULATION OF
INITIAL BOLUS INSULIN DOSE

1. Reduce total current daily prepump insulin by 25%

2. Using the reduced insulin requirement, give:

    • 50% as basal

    • 50% as bolus, divided by 3 and given premeal for 3 meals of equal carbohydrate content

For example:

   Prepump insulin dose = 60 U/day

   CSII requirement = .75 x 60 = 45 U/day

   Basal rate = .5 x 45 = 23 U/day (1 U/h)

   Total bolus dose = .5 x 45 = 23 U/day in 3 equal premeal boluses (7 units before each meal)

Testing the Initial Bolus Dose

Testing and adjustment of the initial bolus dose are based on the blood glucose level four to five hours after the meal, i.e., the next premeal or bedtime blood glucose. These blood glucose measurements should consistently fall within the pump user's individualized target range. Typically, the adjustment is made as follows:

- If the blood glucose is above the target range for two consecutive days at the same time of the day, the preceding premeal bolus is increased on the third and subsequent days by one unit.

- If the blood glucose is below the target range, the preceding premeal bolus is decreased by one unit on subsequent days.

This protocol is repeated until the blood glucose is consistently in the target range. In the event that a change in bolus insulin is repeatedly required, with carbohydrate intake remaining constant, the pump user should be aware that a significant change in activity level, illness, or response to other stress may be responsible. These factors should be evaluated, modified or corrected. If there are no complicating factors and the boluses become grossly disproportionate during this initial phase of equal carbohydrate meals, (e.g. the breakfast bolus is much greater than the lunch bolus), the basal rate should be reevaluated for accuracy (See Chapter 5, *Establishing & Verifying Basal Rates*).

Determining Premeal Boluses Based on the Carbohydrate/Insulin Ratio

When blood glucose levels have been in the target or near-target range for several weeks, the pump user is introduced to adjusting the size of meal boluses based on the grams of carbohydrate to be consumed. This individualized approach greatly increases the flexibility in the timing of meals and the addition of snacks, as well as in the choice of foods eaten, without adversely affecting blood glucose control.

To determine premeal boluses, the grams of carbohydrate in the meal or snack are estimated. Information on the carbohydrate content of various foods may be found on food labels, in books, or by weighing foods on a gram scale and calculating the carbohydrate content from standardized tables. (For more details, refer to Chapter 7, *Counting Carbohydrates*.)

The number of grams of carbohydrate covered by one unit of regular insulin is referred to as the carbohydrate/insulin ratio. This ratio is calculated by dividing the total grams of carbohydrate consumed in a day by the total bolus insulin taken in a day (see Table 2). A dietitian can assist the pump user in calculating an accurate carbohydrate/insulin ratio. The carbohydrate/insulin ratio is typically in the range of 10 to 15 (i.e., 10 to 15 grams of carbohydrate per unit of insulin).

Testing and adjustment of the initial bolus dose are based on the blood glucose level four to five hours after the meal

Table 2

EXAMPLE CALCULATION OF CARBOHYDRATE/INSULIN RATIO

	CHO (grams)	Insulin (units)
Breakfast	110	7.0
Lunch	90	6.0
Dinner	140	10.0
TOTAL	340	23.0

Carbohydrate/Insulin Ratio (340/23) = 15 g/U

Variation in the carbohydrate/insulin ratio from person to person is largely determined by insulin sensitivity. An individual's sensitivity to insulin, in turn, is affected primarily by relative obesity: the more overweight the person, the greater his or her resistance to insulin. An overweight person who is extremely insulin-resistant may have a carbohydrate/insulin ratio of 5/1; that is, he or she may require one unit of insulin for every 5 grams of carbohydrate. Conversely, a very thin, insulin-sensitive person may use only one unit of insulin for every 20 grams of carbohydrate (20/1). If obesity or leanness is not obvious and the carbohydrate/insulin ratio differs significantly from the average of 10 to 15, the variation may be due to inappropriate basal dosing or consistently erroneous carbohydrate counting.

An individual may handle carbohydrate differently at different times of the day, which will cause the carbohydrate/insulin ratio to vary. One unit of insulin often covers fewer grams of carbohydrate at breakfast than it does at other meals. This within-day variation is thought to occur for several reasons:

1. Many persons with diabetes exhibit a "dawn phenomenon," which increases insulin resistance and insulin requirements in the morning (7).

2. Excess premeal boluses taken earlier in the day may affect those taken later, perhaps due to the binding of insulin to antibodies and its delayed release from those antibodies (8).

3. The general activity level may vary significantly over the course of the day.

Typically, these conditions can more consistently be dealt with by adjusting basal insulin rather than by varying the carbohydrate/insulin ratio.

Although carbohydrate has the greatest impact on blood glucose levels and is the usual basis for determining bolus size, it is important to remember that fats and protein can also affect blood glucose and insulin requirements. Fats change the rates of absorption and digestion of carbohydrate. Protein eaten in large quantities can significantly raise blood glucose values over several hours. Bolusing for protein is not generally needed, as protein's contribution to the glycemic effect of food is relatively minor at usual intake levels. An experienced pump user, however, may find the need for a larger than usual bolus before or after a particular meal [for example, the "double-cheese pizza factor" (9)] or use a temporary basal rate for two to three hours to cover a meal high in protein or fat (i.e., square-wave bolus).

Verifying Boluses Based on the Carbohydrate/Insulin Ratio

The beginning carbohydrate/insulin ratio is an estimated value that must be verified for accuracy in each individual. This should be done after the basal insulin profile has been established and verified (see Chapter 5, *Establishing & Verifying Basal Insulin Rates*), and should be repeated periodically to ensure that it remains accurate. A premeal bolus based on a correct ratio returns the blood glucose level to the target range approximately five hours after eating. A typical protocol for testing premeal boluses based on the carbohydrate/insulin ratio is shown below.

Figure 1

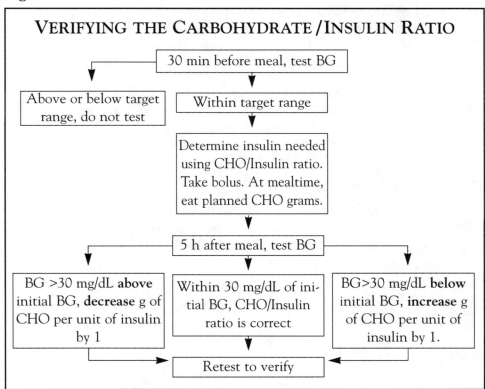

VERIFYING THE CARBOHYDRATE/INSULIN RATIO

30 min before meal, test BG

Above or below target range, do not test

Within target range

Determine insulin needed using CHO/Insulin ratio. Take bolus. At mealtime, eat planned CHO grams.

5 h after meal, test BG

BG >30 mg/dL **above** initial BG, **decrease** g of CHO per unit of insulin by 1

Within 30 mg/dL of initial BG, CHO/Insulin ratio is correct

BG >30 mg/dL **below** initial BG, **increase** g of CHO per unit of insulin by 1.

Retest to verify

Timing of Premeal Boluses

Although the correct carbohydrate/insulin ratio is critical to good glycemic control, another important factor is the timing of the bolus dose before the meal. Typically, the bolus is given 30 minutes before eating to ensure insulin availability during food absorption (1-3). A major cause of postprandial hyperglycemia is failure to deliver the bolus an appropriate length of time before eating.

Bolus timing may be altered depending on the premeal blood glucose level. The pump user can determine the proper amount and timing of a premeal bolus using the following protocol:

1. Check the blood glucose 30 minutes before a meal.

2. Determine the bolus size from the carbohydrate/insulin ratio.

3. If blood glucose is in target range, give bolus and eat 30 minutes later.

4. If blood glucose is low, give the bolus and eat immediately, taking the carbohydrate-containing portion of the meal first. Do not give bolus if food is unavailable. Instead, take a fast-acting carbohydrate to bring the blood glucose level into the target range.

5. If the blood glucose is high (>150 mg/dL), give the bolus 45 minutes, rather than 30 minutes, before the meal. If the blood glucose is above 200 mg/dL, give the bolus 60 minutes before eating (2,10). Delaying the meal permits sufficient insulin absorption to reduce hepatic glucose release and limit the peak postprandial glucose excursion (11). It may not always be practical for the pump user to delay a meal; an alternative approach is eat the carbohydrate portion of the meal later.

As a rule of thumb, the effect of a bolus generally lasts for five to six hours. Therefore, the pump user should be cautious about the possibility of overlapping boluses if administering insulin at shorter intervals than every five hours.

SUPPLEMENTAL INSULIN: COUNTERACTING HIGH BLOOD GLUCOSE LEVELS

In order to safely reduce elevated blood glucose levels, an individual must be aware of his or her insulin sensitivity. The sensitivity factor is defined as the number of mg/dL the blood glucose level typically drops over a two-to four-hour period following administration of one unit of regular insulin. Once this factor is calculated, corrective supplemental doses can be estimated. Different methods can be used to estimate a person's sensitivity factor; the method used in our center is described here.

A major cause of postprandial hyperglycemia is failure to deliver the bolus an appropriate length of time before eating.

The "1500 Rule" (Sensitivity Factor)

The estimated drop in a person's blood glucose per unit of regular insulin can be determined from the following relationship, known as the "1500 Rule." The derived value is referred to as the **sensitivity factor:**

1500/Current Total Daily Insulin Dose = Sensitivity Factor

This relationship was developed as a guideline for devising an individual algorithm for adjusting insulin doses to correct for high blood glucose levels.

It had previously been advised that one unit of supplemental insulin should be given for each 30 mg/dL elevation above the target blood glucose level (4). This relationship, however, was observed to apply only to a person of average size on average doses of insulin, i.e., the 70 kg subject on 50 U/day insulin. The very small person on 10 U/day or the obese, insulin-resistant person on 100 U/day had a different response to supplemental doses of insulin. Their responses supported the presence of an inverse relationship between the total insulin required to maintain target blood glucose levels and the effect of one unit of insulin on the blood glucose.

It was then deduced that the total insulin requirement and the response to one unit of insulin are inversely related in most persons with IDDM. That is, the more total insulin required by the individual, the less the effect of one unit of insulin on the blood glucose level. For example: If a person requiring 50 U/day can anticipate a 30 mg/dL response to one unit of insulin, then the person requiring 30 U/day might expect more of an effect from each unit of insulin, perhaps a 50 mg/dL change in blood glucose. This deduction led to the "1500 Rule" expressed as:

Total insulin per day (50) x blood glucose change per unit (30) = 1500

After 15 years of use as an initial guide to supplemental insulin dosing in a practice of 10,000 persons with diabetes, the "1500 Rule" has proven to be a valuable expedient to initiating a sliding-scale guide for the individualization of insulin therapy. Individuals with a lower sensitivity factor (higher insulin requirements) typically achieve a smaller reduction in blood glucose per unit of insulin than those with a higher sensitivity factor (lower insulin requirements).

The Sensitivity Factor equals 1500 divided by the current total daily insulin dose

SENSITIVITY FACTOR*
(1500/Total Daily Dose)

Current Total Daily Insulin Dose (U)	Sensitivity Factor (mg/dL)
10	150
20	80
25	60
30	50
40	40
50	30
60	25
75	20
100	15
150	10

Estimated reduction in blood glucose per unit of regular insulin based on the total daily insulin dose.

CASE STUDIES: SENSITIVITY FACTORS

1. John W. weighs 160 pounds and enjoys exercising moderately three to four times per week. His total daily insulin requirement averages 26 units. Based on the 1500 Rule, his sensitivity factor is approximately 60:

$$1500/26 = 58 \text{ mg/dL}$$

John can expect a drop of approximately 60 mg/dL in his blood glucose per unit of insulin.

2. Leslie G. weighs 140 pounds and is a full-time student. She walks around campus daily, but spends many hours a day in class and studying. She takes an average of 48 units of insulin per day, making her sensitivity factor approximately 30:

$$1500/48 = 31 \text{ mg/dL}$$

Leslie can predict a drop in blood glucose of 30 mg/dL per unit of insulin.

3. Ray M. weighs 225 pounds and enjoys playing cards in his spare time. He rarely exercises. Ray takes an average of 75 units of insulin per day, making his sensitivity factor approximately 20:

$$1500/75 = 20 \text{ mg/dL}$$

Ray can predict a drop in blood glucose of 20 mg/dL per unit of insulin.

Case	Insulin Requirement	Sensitivity Factor
1	26 units/day	High: 60 mg/dL decrease per unit
2	48 units/day	Average: 30 mg/dL decrease per unit
3	75 units/day	Low: 20 mg/dL decrease per unit

Calculating the Supplemental Insulin Dose

The sensitivity factor is used to calculate an individual's supplemental bolus dose as follows:

$$\text{Supplemental Dose} = (\text{Actual BG - Goal BG})/\text{Sensitivity Factor}$$

where the actual blood glucose is the measured value and the goal blood glucose represents the middle of the person's individualized, premeal target range.

Supplemental insulin is generally given for any elevated blood glucose level occurring before a meal. This insulin is given in addition to the conventional premeal bolus. Should the premeal blood glucose level be lower than the goal blood glucose, the supplemental dose formula is used to reduce the scheduled premeal bolus.

Verifying and Adjusting the Sensitivity Factor

The sensitivity factor is correct if a supplemental dose returns a person's high blood glucose to the target range at the next routine premeal or bedtime check. If, following a supplemental dose, the next routine blood glucose check reveals an unexplained high blood glucose (greater than 180 mg/dL), the pump user should correct the elevation with a further supplemental dose and confirm that the infusion system is working properly. If no infusion-related problems are found, the pump user should verify the accuracy of his or her sensitivity factor using a protocol such as the one shown in Figure 2. For simplicity of calculating supplemental insulin doses, the sensitivity factor is adjusted up or down by increments of ten.

The sensitivity factor can be affected by any condition that alters the total daily insulin requirement. Infection, DKA, renal failure, reaction to glucocorticoid drugs, or a marked change in weight or physical activity may affect blood glucose levels and, therefore, the insulin required for normoglycemia.

In the absence of such complicating factors, the expected reduction in blood glucose brought about by one unit of insulin should remain stable. If the decrease per unit varies greatly from one time of day to another, the basal rate(s) should be retested for accuracy (see Chapter 5, *Establishing & Verifying Basal Insulin Rates*). If the basal rate is correct, and there is a significant change (greater than 20 percent) in the total daily amount of insulin required over a period of five to seven days, the sensitivity factor should be recalculated from the 1500 Rule using the **new** insulin total. Recalculation of the sensitivity factor can be facilitated by retrieving from the pump's memory data on the last week's total insulin delivery.

SPECIAL CONSIDERATIONS

Premeal bolus or supplemental insulin delivery may need to be adjusted under any of the following conditions:

Uncertain Meal Timing or Carbohydrate Content of Meal

"Pulsed" or divided boluses may be necessary if the timing of a meal is uncertain or when the carbohydrate content of a meal is not known, as may be the case when eating at a restaurant. If the meal will be extended, the individual should check his or her blood glucose level approximately 30 minutes before the meal

Recalculation of the sensitivity factor can be facilitated by retrieving from the pump's memory data on the last week's total insulin delivery.

How to Calculate a Supplemental Insulin Dose

The basic formula for calculating a supplemental insulin dose is:

Supplement = (BG-Y)/X, where

BG = Actual blood glucose

Y = Ideal blood glucose (mid-target)

X = Sensitivity Factor (decrease in blood glucose per unit, based on the 1500 Rule)

This formula is used to determine a supplement for a **high blood glucose** as well as for a **low premeal blood glucose.**

Example 1: Positive Supplement

A person with an insulin requirement of 60 units per day and a target BG range of 70-150 mg/dL has a premeal BG of 160.

BG = 160

Y = 100 (target level)

X = 1500/60 = approximately 25

Supplement = (160 - 100)/25 = 2.4 units

The supplement of 2.4 units is given **in addition** to the premeal bolus which is based on the carbohydrate content of the meal.

Example 2: Negative Supplement

A person with an insulin requirement of 60 units per day and a target BG range of 70-150 mg/dL has a premeal BG of 60.

BG = 60

Y = 100

X = 1500/60 = approximately 25

Supplement = (60 - 100)/25 = -1.6 units

In this case, 1.6 units would be **subtracted** from the premeal bolus.

---

is anticipated. If the blood glucose is above the target range, a supplemental insulin dose plus a bolus to cover the appetizer or first course should be taken. When the meal is served, more insulin is taken for any additional carbohydrate that will be eaten. Additional insulin may also be taken at the end of the meal if more carbohydrate than anticipated was eaten. This method allows the pump user to bring blood glucose into target range and helps reduce the concern of developing excessive hyperglycemia or hypoglycemia when the meal timing is beyond control. The pump user should review the time and size of the last two or three meal boluses in the pump's memory in order to avoid overbolusing.

Sick Day Management

A simple illness such as a cold, the flu, or an infection can quickly cause increased blood glucose levels. If no ketones are present, the person should discontinue meals and use supplemental doses every four hours until the blood glucose is <200 mg/dL. If ketones are present, a supplement is given every two hours, without meals, until the blood glucose is near target and ketones are improving. For more details on sick days see Chapter 9, *Everyday Management*.

Figure 2

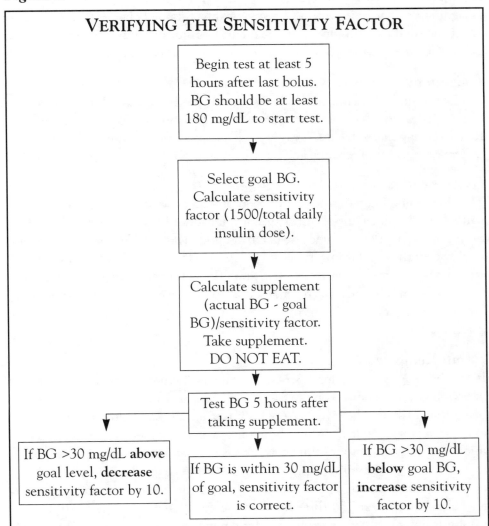

VERIFYING THE SENSITIVITY FACTOR

Begin test at least 5 hours after last bolus. BG should be at least 180 mg/dL to start test.

Select goal BG. Calculate sensitivity factor (1500/total daily insulin dose).

Calculate supplement (actual BG - goal BG)/sensitivity factor. Take supplement. DO NOT EAT.

Test BG 5 hours after taking supplement.

If BG >30 mg/dL **above** goal level, **decrease** sensitivity factor by 10.

If BG is within 30 mg/dL of goal, sensitivity factor is correct.

If BG >30 mg/dL **below** goal BG, **increase** sensitivity factor by 10.

Exercise

A lowering of the blood glucose level is a normal response to exercise. Use of a pump allows the individual to change available insulin levels quickly and efficiently by reducing premeal boluses before exercise or by temporarily lowering the basal rate. Reducing premeal boluses is ideal for moderate or strenuous exercise that occurs within two hours after eating. More detailed information about the effect of exercise on boluses can be found in Chapter 10, *Exercise and the Pump.*

Significant Change in Weight or Activity Level

A significant change in weight or a significant, sustained change in activity may affect the total daily insulin requirement and sensitivity to insulin. Basal rate(s), premeal boluses and supplemental doses may need to be reevaluated.

Pregnancy

Insulin requirements constantly change during pregnancy, which necessitates ongoing adjustment of basal rates, premeal boluses, and supplemental doses. Refer to Chapter 13, *Pump Therapy in Preconception and Pregnancy,* for more information about pregnancy and its effects on insulin requirements.

Gastroparesis

The slowed and unpredictable absorption of food associated with gastroparesis will affect glycemic control. If this condition cannot be moderated with medications such as metoclopramide (Reglan), cisapride (Propulside), or erythromycin, then the effect of bolus insulin must be delayed. This may be accomplished by eliminating pre-meal boluses, as such, and using a higher, temporary basal rate for three hours after meals. This method allows the increased insulin effect to be spread over a period of several hours, reducing the risk for postprandial hypoglycemia.

Pump Removal

It may become necessary for a person to temporarily suspend pump use. For brief periods of pump removal (one to four hours), the amount of regular insulin not being infused should be given as a bolus injection. For more prolonged periods of pump removal, regular insulin should be given every four to five hours by injection. (This necessitates interrupting sleep to avoid overnight loss of control.) The injected insulin dose should include: 1) the usual premeal bolus based on carbohydrate intake, 2) any supplement necessary to compensate for the current blood glucose, and 3) three hours of the usual basal rate. Use of NPH insulin is not generally recommended for temporary periods of pump removal; if NPH is used, dosages need to be individually established. In all cases of pump removal, careful blood glucose monitoring should guide any adjustments.

Divided boluses may be necessary if the timing of a meal is uncertain or when the carbohydrate content of a meal is not known, as may be the case when eating at a restaurant.

SUMMARY

Use of an insulin pump provides precise and efficient delivery of bolus and supplemental insulin tailored to meet the individual's own needs. Carbohydrate counting and use of the carbohydrate/insulin ratio permit accurate calculation of premeal bolus doses, which should be delivered at least 30 minutes before eating to allow for insulin absorption from the subcutaneous tissue. Calculation of accurate supplemental insulin doses is facilitated through use of the sensitivity factor. Together with correctly established basal rates, these tools give the person with insulin-dependent diabetes the means to achieve optimal glycemic control.

For more prolonged periods of pump removal, regular insulin should be given every four to five hours by injection.

REFERENCES

1. Lauritzen T, Pramming S, Deckert T, Binder C. Pharmacokinetics of continuous subcutaneous insulin infusion. *Diabetologia* 1983;24:326-329.

2. Dimitriadis GD, Gerich JE. Importance of timing of preprandial subcutaneous insulin administration in the management of diabetes mellitus. *Diabetes Care* 1983;6:374-377.

3. Kinmonth AL, Baum JD. Timing of pre-breakfast insulin injection and postprandial metabolic control in diabetic children. *Br Med J* 1980;604-606.

4. Skyler JS, Seigler DE, Reeves ML. Optimizing pumped insulin delivery. *Diabetes Care* 1982;5:135-139.

5. Chantelau E, Sonnenberg GE, Stanitzek-Schmidt I, Best F, Altenhr H, Berger M. Diet liberalization and metabolic control in type I diabetic outpatients treated by continuous subcutaneous insulin infusion. *Diabetes Care* 1982;5:612-616.

6. Grinvalsky M, Nathan DM. Diets for insulin pump and multiple daily injection therapy. *Diabetes Care* 1983;6:241-244.

7. Koivisto VA, Yki-Jarvinen H, Helve E, Karonen S-L, Pelkonen R. Pathogenesis and prevention of the dawn phenomenon in diabetic patients treated with CSII. *Diabetes* 1986;35:78-82.

8. Zinman B. The physiologic replacement of insulin. *N Engl J Med* 1989;321:363-370.

9. Ahern J, Garcomb PM, Held NA, Petit WA, Tamborlane WV. Exaggerated hyperglycemia after a pizza meal in well-controlled diabetes. *Diabetes Care* 1993;16:578-580.

10. Witt MF, White NH, Santiago JV. Roles of site and timing of the morning insulin injection in type I diabetes. *J Pediat* 1983;103:528-533.

11. Farkas-Hirsch R, Levandoski LA. Implementation of continuous subcutaneous insulin infusion therapy: an overview. *Diabetes Educ* 1986;14:401-406.

12. Barnett JL, Vinik AI. Gastrointestinal disturbances. In: Lebovitz HE, ed. *Therapy for Diabetes Mellitus and Related Disorders*, Second Edition. Alexandria, VA: American Diabetes Association; 1994:289-292.

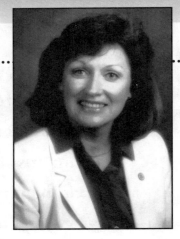

BETTY PAGE BRACKENRIDGE, MS, RD, CDE

Betty Brackenridge, a past president of the American Association of Diabetes Educators, is well known as a writer and speaker for both lay and professional diabetes audiences. She has a special interest in nutrition for intensive diabetes therapy and has long been an advocate of carbohydrate counting because of its accuracy and simplicity. Both a registered dietitian and a certified diabetes educator, Betty received her Master of Science in Human Nutrition from Arizona State University in Tempe. In recent years, her work has extended to the international arena where she presents workshops in educational methods to health care providers of all disciplines. Her first book, *Diabetes 101*, is used as the text for diabetes education classes in many hospitals and outpatient centers. Her next book, *Sweet Kids*, to be published by the American Diabetes Association in 1996, explores how the nutritional demands of diabetes can be managed in the context of healthy family relationships.

JOHN HAMILTON "CHIP" REED, MD

Dr. Reed is an endocrinologist in private practice with Northside Endocrinology in Atlanta, Georgia. He is also an Associate Clinical faculty member at Emory University and a Medical Director for the State of Georgia Diabetes Camp. He has a special interest in carbohydrates and promoting the use of carbohydrate counting to optimize diabetes management.

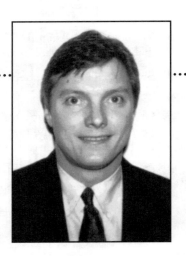

Counting Carbohydrates 7

THE KEY TO PROPER BOLUSING

Nutrition is an essential component of successful diabetes management. Proper nutrition aids glycemic control and supplies the nutrients needed for overall good health. Frequent blood glucose testing and the right meal planning approach are necessary to ensure that nutritional goals are being met and that the pump user is getting maximum benefit from the insulin pump's capabilities. For ideal glycemic control, the pump user should have a meal planning approach that is as precise and flexible as the pump. Counting carbohydrate is one of the most precise and adaptable ways to manage meals (1-3). It is easy to learn and use, and when the pump user is adept at it, carbohydrate counting can add a lot of freedom to food choices.

Carbohydrate (starches and sugars) accounts for most of the glucose in the bloodstream, especially right after meals. In fact, 90 to 100 percent of the digestible starches and sugars eaten appear in the blood as glucose within a few hours after they are consumed. Carbohydrate, as starches and sugars, is found in:

- Fruits and vegetables
- Starchy vegetables, like potatoes and corn
- Grain products, like bread, crackers, cookies, rice, cereal, and pasta
- Dried or canned beans, peas, and lentils
- Dairy products, particularly milk and yogurt
- Sugar and sugar-sweetened foods

Carbohydrate counting allows the pump user to calculate the premeal bolus dose of insulin based on the actual amount of carbohydrate to be eaten.

IN THIS CHAPTER

Counting Methods

Reading Food Labels

Glycemic Index

Maintaining Weight

Handling Alcohol

METHODS OF COUNTING CARBOHYDRATE

The two main methods of counting carbohydrate, summarized in the table below, differ in their degree of simplicity and precision. The best method for a given individual is the one that is easiest to use and that produces the desired level of blood glucose control.

The first method involves the use of exchanges or *carbs* (15-gram carbohydrate portions) to count carbohydrates. Using *carbs* has several advantages: it is simple, it builds on knowledge the pump user may already have, and, because it requires working with smaller numbers, it can reduce the chance for math errors. However, it may not be precise enough to achieve blood glucose goals in all individuals. The more precise carbohydrate gram counting method takes more effort and math skill. In general, the smaller the individual's body size and the more insulin-sensitive he or she is, the more likely the precision of carbohydrate gram counting will be required.

In general, the smaller the individual's body size and the more insulin-sensitive he or she is, the more likely the precision of carbohydrate gram counting will be required.

Method	Description	Bolus Calculation	Ease vs. Accuracy
Counting *Carbs* or Exchanges	• Count servings of Starch/Bread, Fruit, and Milk, considering them all to be equal in carb value (15 grams/*carb*). • Vegetables contain 1/3 *carb* per serving. (Not counted by some clinicians.) • Meat/Protein is not usually counted (However, if it is, assume about 1/3 *carb* per ounce or exchange).	Calculate bolus as units of insulin per *carb*	• Easiest method but also the least precise. • Requires little math skill and uses exchange groups and portions, which the pump user may already know.
Counting Grams of Carbohydrate	• Add carbohydrate gram values for all foods eaten to obtain carbohydrate total for meal. • If counting the glucose value of protein (not required for most individuals), multiply grams of protein in meal by 0.6 to estimate available glucose, and add to grams of carbohydrate.	Calculate bolus by dividing the total grams of carbohydrate in a meal by the carbohydrate-to-insulin ratio (*See Chapter 6*).	• Very accurate but more time-consuming than counting carbs. • Requires some math skill to add and divide 2- and 3-digit numbers, especially if done mentally.

Counting Exchanges or Carbs

Food exchange lists assign an average carbohydrate value per exchange to all the foods in each food group:

- Starches/Breads = 15 grams = 1 *carb*
- Fruits = 15 grams = 1*carb*
- Milk = 12 grams = 1 *carb*
- Vegetables = 5 grams = 1/3 *carb*
- Fats = 0 grams = 0 *carb*
- Meat/Proteins = 0 grams

To count *carbs*, the pump user counts servings of Starch/Bread, Fruit, and Milk, considering them all to be equal in *carb* value (about 15 grams per *carb*). Vegetables contain an average of 1/3 *carb* per serving. Not all clinicians require individuals to count this source of carbohydrate. However, if the patient consumes more than 1 to 2 servings per meal, better glucose control may be achieved by counting vegetables.

With the *carb*-counting system, the bolus insulin dose is calculated as units per *carb* (15-gram portion), based on the pump user's sensitivity to insulin. The starting bolus is usually based on one unit per *carb*, and is adjusted up or down in 0.5 unit increments (or 0.1 unit increments, for more insulin-sensitive pump users) until glycemic goals are achieved.

Because exchange values are averages, they are not accurate for every food in a group. On a single item, the difference isn't large enough to make a difference in the bolus dose calculation. But when the carbohydrate content of a whole meal is estimated using exchanges, there may be a big difference between the exchange estimate and the actual value. The pump user should use blood glucose levels as a guide. If glycemic goals are not being met, the pump user should be advised to try the more precise carbohydrate gram counting method.

Counting Carbohydrate Grams

In carbohydrate gram counting, the pump user adds the carbohydrate gram values for all foods eaten to obtain the carbohydrate total for a meal. Carbohydrate gram values can be obtained from reliable food lists, reference books, and food product nutrition labels. In fact, counting carbohydrate grams is greatly simplified by the ready availability of food product Nutrition Facts labels.

With this approach, the premeal bolus insulin dose is calculated by dividing the total grams of carbohydrate in the meal by the carbohydrate/insulin ratio, as explained in Chapter 6, *Bolus & Supplemental Insulin*.

Counting carbohydrate grams is greatly simplified by the ready availability of food product Nutrition Facts labels.

SOURCES OF INFORMATION

Food Labels

Most packaged and processed foods have nutrition information labels. The label lists the number of calories, the grams of carbohydrate, protein, and fat in a specified serving size of the food, as well as other information. The following is a sample label, showing the Nutrition Facts for a frozen chicken and rice dinner:

Most people with diabetes can estimate the appropriate bolus dose for any meal or snack simply by counting carbohydrate content.

Nutrition Facts

Frozen Chicken & Rice Dinner
Serving Size 1 box

Amount per Serving

Calories 356	Calories from Fat 72

	% Daily Value
Total Fat 8g	13%
Saturated Fat 4g	7%
Cholesterol 0mg	0%
Sodium 567 mg	25%
Total Carbohydrate 45g	14%
Dietary Fiber 3g	12%
Sugars 0g	0%
Protein 26g	

For those counting *carbs* or exchanges, the carbohydrate gram value listed on the label is divided by 15 to find the number of *carbs* provided by one serving.

For carbohydrate gram counting, the listed carbohydrate values can be used as is, or can be adjusted, if necessary, for the effects of dietary fiber. Because the fiber content of the food is not digested and thus contributes no glucose, using the total carbohydrate value can cause an overestimation of the amount of glucose yielded by high-fiber foods (those that contain more than five grams of fiber per serving). Therefore, if boluses calculated using the total carbohydrate content of high-fiber foods do not produce the desired degree of glycemic control, the grams of dietary fiber can be subtracted from the total carbohydrate to find a more precise value.

Food Composition Lists and Books

Lists of the nutrient content of some common foods can be found in publications available in the "Nutrition and Diet" section of bookstores and libraries. Excellent references include *Food Value of Portions Commonly Used,* by

Pennington and Church (Harper, Collins Publisher), and *The Complete Book of Food Counts,* 3rd Edition, by Corrinne Netzer (Dell Publishing). Similar books are available that list the nutrient content of many convenience and restaurant foods such as *Fast Food Facts* by Marion Franz (ChroniMed Publishing). There are also books that list only the carbohydrate content of foods, such as Barbara Krause's *Guide To Carbohydrates* (New American Library).

CARBOHYDRATE AND THE GLYCEMIC INDEX

Counting carbohydrate is simple and it works, but it is not a perfect system. Research indicates that not all carbohydrates are created equal when it comes to their effect on blood glucose. That is, foods differ in their "glycemic index" or their ability to raise the blood glucose level (4-6). For example, a serving of plain boiled potatoes has been shown to raise the blood glucose higher than an equal sized serving of baked potatoes (7). Carbohydrate from corn flakes usually raises blood glucose higher and more quickly than an equal dose from table sugar. These differences are caused chiefly by how quickly the carbohydrates from different foods are digested and absorbed.

The glycemic index of a food relates to whether a particular food will cause the blood glucose to "spike" in the first couple of hours after eating. Low glycemic index foods release their glucose to the bloodstream slowly. High glycemic index foods release theirs all at once. However, this does not necessarily mean that the premeal bolus should change with the glycemic index of the foods eaten. For example, for most people, a food like mashed potatoes, which has a high glycemic index, can be expected to raise the blood glucose higher and more quickly than *al dente* pasta, which has a lower glycemic index. If the blood glucose is 100 mg/dL before supper, and an equal number of grams of carbohydrate from either potatoes or pasta, eaten in a mixed meal, is covered with a correct insulin bolus, the bedtime blood glucose value should approximate 100 mg/dL in either case. The only question remaining is whether the one or two hour postmeal blood glucose elevation produced by the high glycemic index food is acceptable to the pump user. If it is not, several strategies are available to prevent an elevated postmeal blood glucose:

- Choosing a lower glycemic index food or adding some fat to the higher glycemic index choice (such as having margarine on the mashed potatoes)
- Increasing the fiber in the meal by having a raw vegetable or bean salad, instead of lettuce, to slow down digestion and absorption
- Waiting longer to eat after taking the premeal bolus to achieve a better match between the glucose and insulin profiles

With experience and through routine monitoring of blood glucose, a pump user can discover the effect that specific foods and meals have on his or her own blood glucose level.

The glycemic index is not a precise tool. Although the relative differences between foods are known, their exact effect on blood glucose differs significantly among individuals. It may be further affected by the amount of fat and protein in the meal, the amount and type of fiber in the meal, how fast and in what order the foods are eaten, and whether the carbohydrate is eaten raw or cooked. With experience and through routine monitoring of blood glucose, a pump user can discover the effect that specific foods and meals have on his or her own blood glucose level, and be better able to make decisions about food choices, portions, and bolus doses and timing that will result in the best possible control.

DERIVING THE CARBOHYDRATE COUNTING MEAL PLAN

The basic meal plan for an individual who uses carbohydrate counting is composed of gram totals for the amount of carbohydrate to be consumed at each planned meal and snack. There are two ways to develop such a plan. The preferred method is to base the plan on the person's current eating habits. An average or usual meal pattern can be identified using several days of food records provided by the pump user. This pattern can then be translated into the carbohydrate gram equivalent consumed at each meal or snack. Any desirable changes to improve overall nutritional intake or to address specific risk factors can be negotiated on an incremental basis as education progresses.

Alternatively, a carbohydrate plan can be derived from an estimated or calculated calorie prescription by multiplying the caloric intake by the desired proportion of carbohydrate and dividing the resulting value by four. For example, a person is estimated to require 2000 calories and the goal is for him or her to consume 50 percent of calories as carbohydrate. Multiply 2000 kilocalories by 0.5 and divide the resulting value (1000) by 4 kilocalories per gram of carbohydrate. The total daily carbohydrate allowance would be 250 grams. This total allowance is then distributed among the day's meals and snacks with attention to the pump user's preferences for meal size and composition.

When the meal plan is developed in this fashion, the calculated carbohydrate allowance must be compared to the pump user's current intake. Care should be taken to minimize dramatic differences between the calculated carbohydrate allowance and the actual intake since current insulin doses were undoubtedly derived in association with the customary carbohydrate intake. Insulin doses may need to be altered to prevent loss of glucose control if large changes are made in the calorigenic composition of the diet.

The basic meal plan should be followed fairly closely for the first month or so, while the pump user learns the carbohydrate counting system and stabilizes diabetes control. A stable food intake makes it much easier to correctly adjust the basal insulin rates and, later, to accurately derive the person's

The basic meal plan should be followed fairly closely for the first month or so, while the pump user learns the carbohydrate counting system and stabilizes diabetes control.

carbohydrate/insulin ratio (refer to Chapter 6). When this ratio is known, the pump user can match insulin doses to actual food intake in order to accommodate variations in appetite, food availability, personal or work circumstances and other factors.

CAN PROTEIN EFFECT BLOOD GLUCOSE?

The exact effects of carbohydrate, fats, and protein depend on several factors, including digestion, absorption, fuel mix, and overall composition of the meal, and can vary significantly from person to person (4, 8-12). However, most people with diabetes can estimate the appropriate bolus dose for any meal or snack simply by counting carbohydrate content. Because some individuals appear to get better results when they account for protein as well, it is included here for discussion.

Several sources suggest that 50 to 70 percent of protein can be deaminated and converted to glucose under certain conditions (9, 10, 13). However, few controlled studies in diabetic persons have been done to confirm or quantify the specific effects of protein on blood glucose levels in this population. Still, it appears clinically that protein may have a noticeable effect on glucose in certain individuals. The apparent effect of protein on blood glucose seem to occur some hours after eating.

It appears that when protein intake falls within nutritional guidelines (10 to 20 percent of total calories) and is consistent from day to day, the insulin needs created by protein are met by the basal insulin rate for most people. However, some individuals seem to achieve better blood glucose control when they account for protein in addition to carbohydrate in calculating their insulin bolus doses. This seems to be associated with smaller body size, greater insulin sensitivity or unusually large protein intake, but the particulars of such responses have not been confirmed under controlled circumstances.

However, from a purely pragmatic perspective, if glucose goals are not achieved when calculating boluses by counting only carbohydrate, the possible effect of protein could be tested. This test can be done in one of two ways. The easiest method for most pump users would be to continue consuming their usual meals but to try calculating their boluses including the effect of protein. Suggested methods for including the possible effect of protein are as follows:

- *Carb counting method:* Each Meat/Protein exchange (1 oz.) is counted as 1/3 carb.
- *Carbohydrate gram counting method:* Grams of protein in a meal are multiplied by 0.6 (60 percent). This value is added to the carbohydrate grams to obtain the meal total for "available glucose."

If glucose goals are not achieved when calculating boluses by counting only carbohydrate, the possible effect of protein could be tested.

Since any effect of protein on blood glucose is assumed to occur some hours after eating, the next premeal blood glucose value is a reasonable indicator of the presence of this effect, provided there have been no snacks between the meals. Blood glucose control can then be compared to the period when carbohydrate alone was used to calculate boluses, and the provider and pump user can determine together whether the extra effort is of any value.

MAINTAINING, NOT GAINING

Better blood glucose control and intensive insulin therapy can lead to unwanted weight gain (14). This happens because:

1. As glycemic control improves, glucose calories are no longer lost in the urine.

2. As proper insulin doses are being determined, hypoglycemia may occur more frequently and, consequently, more food may be eaten to counteract it.

3. Confidence in managing diet and insulin may lead to more frequent "splurging" on sweets and other favorite foods.

When glucose control is excellent, the body behaves as it would if diabetes were not present. Consuming more calories than are needed results in weight gain. Pump users should be reminded that 3500 extra calories equals one extra pound. The best way to deal with the problem of weight gain is to stop it before it starts.

If previous blood glucose control has not been very good, consider reducing calorie intake when pump therapy is started. This helps make up for the unused calories that have previously been excreted from the body due to high blood glucose levels. Regular exercise is the best protection against extra pounds, and a pump makes it much easier to manage exercise without hypoglycemia. Fat and alcohol intake should be watched closely. These foods are concentrated sources of calories and add little nutritional value to the diet. Weighing regularly, perhaps every Monday morning, may help to prevent unwanted weight gain. However, if the individual is underweight due to previous poor control when pump therapy is initiated, calorie reduction is probably not indicated, at least until desirable weight and metabolic stability are achieved. If necessary, a dietitian should be consulted for more ideas about how to achieve and maintain desirable weight.

For individuals with IDDM who want to lose weight, pump therapy can facilitate weight loss while decreasing the risk of hypoglycemia. The pump user can safely reduce food intake and make corresponding adjustments in bolus doses, while the basal rate covers the background insulin requirements.

If previous blood glucose control has not been very good, consider reducing calorie intake when pump therapy is started.

CARBOHYDRATE COUNTING AND BOLUSES IN ACTION

Real-life situations often provide the best educational tools in learning to coordinate carbohydrate counting and insulin dosing. The following section includes scenarios that may be familiar.

1. High Blood Glucose After Breakfast
"Even though my control at other times is very good, my blood glucose after breakfast always seems to be high. What might be causing this?"

There are two possible explanations. Either one or both may be contributing to the problem. The first, known as the "dawn phenomenon," is characterized by an increase in the insulin requirement in the early morning hours as a result of an increase in the level of growth hormone. Growth hormone causes increased insulin resistance; that is, it can take more insulin to cover a given amount of carbohydrate early in the morning. Programming a higher basal rate during early morning hours or using a slightly higher ratio of carbohydrate to insulin for breakfast can help control this situation. The other factor that may contribute to high blood glucose levels after breakfast is that most of the foods that tend to be eaten at breakfast are high in carbohydrate: fruits, juices, toast, bagels, pancakes, cereal and so on. The carbohydrate count, based on the portion size, for each food must be as accurate as possible, because even small errors on individual foods can contribute to a large cumulative error for the entire meal. If the carbohydrate estimate is too low, the bolus will be too small, resulting in a high blood glucose level after breakfast. In addition, boluses should be given a sufficient amount of time before the meal (typically 30 minutes or more).

2. Overbolusing For Favorite Foods
"I had a reaction after taking an extra five-unit bolus for a Snickers chocolate bar. What went wrong?"

Estimating the bolus for chocolate candy and other sweets can be tricky. In this situation, it appears that the person overestimated the effect the Snickers Bar would have on the blood glucose. Many people are very aware of the sugar that candy contains and assume it will elevate the blood glucose quite dramatically. However, most sweets are also high in fat, and some contain nuts as well, both of which tend to lower the glycemic effect of whatever sugar the candy contains. In addition, there may not be as much sugar as one might think. A review of the label on the candy bar reveals it contains 36 grams of carbohydrate or *2-1/2 carbs.* Unless there is a need to take 1 unit of insulin for every 7 grams of carbohydrate, the bolus taken was simply too large. Most people would need 2.5 to 3.5 units of regular insulin to cover the Snickers Bar. Determining the correct bolus is often best done through trial and error.

Meal plans for pump users should be based on their current eating habits, with any changes negotiated on a stepwise basis as education progresses.

3. Alcoholic Beverages
"How do I figure out my bolus for alcoholic beverages?

Pure alcohol alone does not raise blood glucose. Therefore, no bolus is needed for the alcohol content of mixed drinks, beer or wine. In fact, **alcohol itself increases the risk for hypoglycemia.** This happens chiefly because the liver cannot make new glucose while it is processing alcohol. This prevents the body's normal protective mechanism from "kicking in" if the blood glucose falls while drinking (15). **Alcohol should never be taken on an empty stomach.** One or two low-carbohydrate alcoholic drinks, such as dry wine, bourbon and water, or gin and diet tonic, can usually be added to a normal meal plan with little effect on the blood glucose. Some alcoholic drinks such as sweet wines, liqueurs, and mixed drinks made with regular soda, syrup or fruit juice (margaritas and screwdrivers) may have carbohydrates that need to be counted. Typically, less insulin is required per gram of carbohydrate when drinking alcohol. Bolusing for carbohydrate when drinking should be done very carefully because of the increased risk of delayed hypoglycemia. Since alcohol can impair reasoning, extra care is called for in calculating bolus insulin doses when drinking. Additional blood glucose testing is required post alcohol consumption to prevent unrecognized hypoglycemia.

SUMMARY

Carbohydrate counting, using either the exchange system (*carbs*) or gram counting, gives pump users the flexibility to plan meals that meet their lifestyle and nutritional goals, and to match meals with precise insulin bolus doses. Some pump users, particularly those who are highly insulin-sensitive, require the precision of carbohydrate gram counting, and may also need to account for the possible effects of protein in calculating total grams of "available glucose" provided by a meal. Meal plans for pump users should be based on their current eating habits, with any changes negotiated on a stepwise basis as education progresses.

REFERENCES

1. Holler HJ, Pastors JG, eds. *Meal Planning Approaches for Diabetes Management.* 2nd ed. Chicago,IL: American Diabetes Association, 1994.

2. Brackenridge BP. Carbohydrate gram counting: a key to accurate mealtime boluses in intensive therapy. *Pract Diabetol* 1992;11:22-28.

3. Pastors JG. Alternatives to the exchange system for teaching meal planning to people with diabetes. *Diabetes Educ* 1992;18:57-62.

4. Jenkins DJ, Wolever TM, Taylor RH, Barker H, Fielden H, Baldwin J, Bowling A, Newman H, Jenkins A, Goff D. Glycemic index of foods: a physiological basis for carbohydrate exchange. *Am J Clin Nutr* 1981;34:184-190.

5. Hollenbeck CB, Coulston AM, Reaven GM. Comparison of plasma glucose and insulin responses to mixed meals of high-, intermediate-, and low-glycemic potential. *Diabetes Care* 1988;11:323-329.

6. Laine DC, Thomas W, Levitt MD, Bantle JP. Comparison of predictive capabilities of diabetic exchange lists and glycemic index of foods. *Diabetes Care* 1987;19:387-394.

7. Lunetta M, DiMauro M, Crioni S, Mughini L. Influence of different cooking processes on the glycemic response to potatoes in non-insulin dependent diabetic patients. *Diab Nutr Metab* 1995;8:49-53.

8. Peters AL, Davidson MB. Protein and fat effects on glucose response and insulin requirements in subjects with insulin-dependent diabetes mellitus. *Am J Clin Nutr* 1993;58:555-560.

9. Nuttall FQ, Mooradien AD, Gannon MC. Effect of protein ingestion on the glucose and insulin response to standardized oral glucose load. *Diabetes Care* 1984,7:465-470.

10. Nuttall FQ, Gannon MC. Plasma glucose and insulin response to macronutrients in nondiabetic and NIDDM subjects. *Diabetes Care* 1991,14:824-834.

11. Choppin J, Jovanovic-Peterson L, Peterson C. Matching food with insulin. *Diabetes Professional* 1991; Spring:1-14.

12. Ahern JA, Gatcomb PM, Held NA, Petit WA, Tamborlane WV. Exaggerated hyperglycemia after a pizza meal in well-controlled diabetes. *Diabetes Care* 1993;16:578-580.

13. Oexmann MJ. *Total Available Glucose, Diabetic Food System*. Charleston, SC: Medical University of South Carolina Printing Service; 1987.

14. DCCT Research Group. Weight gain associated with intensive therapy in the Diabetes Control and Complications Trial. *Diabetes Care* 1988;11:567-573.

15. Avogaro A, Beltramello P, Gnudi L, Maran A, Valerio A, Miola M, Marin N, Cerpaldi C, Confortin L, Costa F, MacDonald I, Tiengo A. Alcohol intake impairs glucose counterregulation during acute insulin-induced hypoglycemia in IDDM patients. *Diabetes* 1993;42:1626-1634.

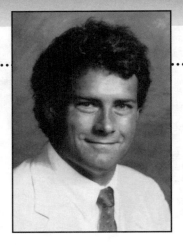

BRUCE W. BODE, MD

An internationally known speaker and author on insulin pump therapy, Dr. Bode is in private practice with the Atlanta Diabetes Associates and serves as Medical Director, Diabetes Treatment Center of America at West Paces Medical Center, Atlanta, GA. He also serves as President of the American Diabetes Association, Georgia Affiliate, and is on the Board of Directors of the Juvenile Diabetes Foundation, Atlanta chapter.

PAUL C. DAVIDSON, MD

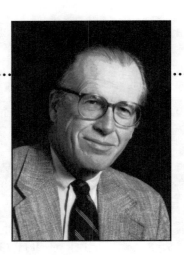

Dr. Davidson is Medical Director of the Diabetes Treatment Center of America at West Paces Ferry Hospital, Atlanta, Georgia, and serves on the DTCA's Medical Advisory Council. He is also a founding partner and private practitioner in Atlanta Diabetes Associates, Atlanta, GA, an endocrinology group practice providing primary and consultative care for persons with diabetes. Dr. Davidson served as Associate Editor of *Annals of Internal Medicine* from 1976 to 1978. A developer of the Glucommander insulin infusion program, Dr. Davidson became a principal investigator for the MiniMed Implantable Pump Program in 1990. He firmly believes in the use of the insulin pump for controlling diabetes – to date, his center has placed over 600 patients on the pump.

PATTERN ANALYSIS & RECORDKEEPING

8

Self-monitoring and recording of blood glucose levels are essential elements in any intensive diabetes management program, including those based on insulin pump therapy. Logical recordkeeping assists both the pump user and the diabetes care team in promptly identifying and correcting patterns of out-of-range blood glucose levels. This chapter addresses some of the important considerations surrounding the use of blood glucose levels in guiding insulin pump therapy.

REGULAR SELF-MONITORING IS ESSENTIAL

Regular self-monitoring of blood glucose (SMBG) helps to ensure the pump user's safety by revealing possibly unsuspected hypo- or hyperglycemia and also permits fine-tuning of basal, bolus, and supplemental insulin doses to guard against out-of-range blood glucose excursions. All pump users should be thoroughly trained in SMBG technique, testing schedules, and recording requirements.

Pump users should monitor blood glucose levels at least four times a day — before each meal, and at bedtime. In addition, they should monitor their blood glucose once a week at 3 AM, or whenever their prebreakfast blood glucose levels are outside of their target range. More frequent monitoring is necessary during illness and when taking prescription drugs that may alter insulin action, decrease awareness of hypoglycemia, or impair glucose counterregulation (1). Self-monitoring is also useful to assess the effect of planned or unplanned changes in activity level or major changes in diet.

Target blood glucose ranges should be individually established. Properly set target levels aid pump users in achieving optimal control, while minimizing the risks for hypoglycemia. Individuals with any of the following conditions require higher glycemic goals than those without such conditions: reduced hypoglycemia awareness, untreatable coronary artery disease, advanced microvascular disease, and learning disabilities (2). Guidelines for setting blood glucose target levels are found in Chapter 5, *Establishing & Verifying Basal Insulin Rates*. Every pump user should know his or her target blood glucose range, and it is recommended that the health care provider write this range at the top of the pump user's recordkeeping sheet.

It is recommended that the health care provider write the target blood glucose range at the top of the pump user's record-keeping sheet.

GLUCOSE METER CALIBRATION

A capillary finger-stick performed and read by the pump user should be compared to a blood glucose determination done by the laboratory in order to validate the individual's testing technique and the instrument's accuracy. This requires that the pump user bring his or her meter to an office visit. The blood glucose level measured in whole blood is 15 percent lower than the laboratory measurement done on plasma or serum.

The American Diabetes Association recommends that an SMBG test system permit a user to achieve a total error of less than 10 percent at glucose concentrations ranging from 30 to 400 mg/dL (1). Health care professionals should carefully review clinical performance data on any SMBG systems (meters plus test strips) they are considering recommending to clients. Test systems that have been shown to yield coefficients of variation <10 percent comply with the stringent ADA consensus guidelines.

DAILY RECORDKEEPING

Logical recordkeeping is essential in any form of intensive insulin therapy. Recordkeeping makes possible the analysis of blood glucose patterns and their association with diet, insulin, activity, and other factors, thereby helping pump users achieve better blood glucose control. In a group of 205 pump users, those who recorded blood glucose levels on a log sheet maintained a significantly lower mean glycosylated hemoglobin (HbA_{1c}) level over the 2.9-year mean study period than those who did not record (7.1 percent vs. 7.9 percent, $p<0.0001$, normal 3.4 to 6.1 percent) (3).

Use of a blood glucose meter with memory can also facilitate recordkeeping and pattern analysis. Various software programs are available for analysis of blood glucose trends using data downloaded from a meter's memory.

Prior to pump initiation, the client and health care professional should review together the data that need to be recorded in order to evaluate the effectiveness of pump therapy. These parameters include blood glucose levels, basal rate changes, boluses, supplemental insulin doses to correct for both high and low blood glucose values, hypoglycemic events with and without symptoms, exercise times, and infusion set changes.

A convenient recordkeeping system that is designed for facsimile (FAX) transmission of all key data facilitates timely communication between the pump user and the diabetes care team. The diabetes care team takes an active role in analyzing patterns of blood glucose levels and related events, gradually turning this responsibility over as the pump user acquires the necessary experience and understanding. During the first month after pump initiation, it is suggested that pump users fax their flow sheets twice a week. When better control is achieved, an individual can reduce the frequency of reporting to weekly or monthly. The provider should ask for more frequent reports if a person requires improved control, becomes slack in self-monitoring, needs psychological reinforcement (e.g., adolescents or adults under stress), or is pregnant.

Shown in Figure 1, the flow sheet has spaces for a full month's worth of data, with one line devoted to each day. There are spaces for all necessary data including blood glucose readings, meal boluses, supplemental insulin doses, up to three basal insulin profiles, hypoglycemic episodes, exercise, weight, and remarks. Arrows link the columns containing blood glucose readings with the columns containing related insulin dosing information, as follows:

- 3 AM blood glucose is affected by basal profile #1
- Prebreakfast blood glucose is affected by basal profile #2
- Prelunch blood glucose is affected by prebreakfast bolus and supplement
- Presupper blood glucose is affected by prelunch bolus and supplement
- Bedtime blood glucose is affected by presupper bolus and supplement

This linkage helps both the provider and the pump user to readily relate out-of-range blood glucose levels to their possible cause. Supplemental doses are recorded separately from premeal boluses to permit analysis of their effect, as illustrated in Case Study #3.

BLOOD GLUCOSE PATTERN ANALYSIS

Upon receipt of a person's flow sheet, we highlight all blood glucose levels outside of his or her target range, using one color highlighter (pink) for low blood glucose levels and another color (yellow) for high levels. (Pump users should be encouraged to mark their own out-of-range levels by drawing circles around low levels and boxes around high levels. Color highlighting does not fax, and tends to obscure the data when it is faxed.)

We highlight all blood glucose levels outside of the pump user's target range, using one color highlighter (pink) for low blood glucose levels and another color (yellow) for high levels.

Figure 1

EXAMPLE BLOOD GLUCOSE FLOW SHEET

Name _____   Doctor _____

Address _____   For Month _____ Year _____

City _____ State _____ Zip _____   Supplemental Formula _____

Phone: Home _____ Work _____   Target Range _____

TIME	3 AM	PRE-BREAKFAST				NOON				PRE-SUPPER			BEDTIME	REMARKS
DATE	Basal Profile 1	BG	Basal Profile 2	BG	REG.	SUP.		BG	REG.	SUP.		BG	REG.	SUP.	BG	* REACTION # EXERCISE RECORD WT. @ WEEKLY
																BASAL BEGIN END
																1ST
																2ND
																3RD

In looking for patterns, we review the data over three days to one week. For longer-term pump users who are under good control, monthly review is usually sufficient. In addition, we check the data from the pump's memory (the last seven boluses and the last week's daily totals) during a visit to verify recordkeeping. The goals of pattern analysis are to help the pump user fine-tune the various insulin dosages (supplemental, bolus, and basal), as well as to identify and correct other possible causes of out-of-range blood glucose levels.

To analyze the accuracy of the supplemental dose, we look for every high blood glucose level and the level immediately following it. Specifically, if every high blood glucose level is followed by one in the target range, this indicates that the patient's supplemental dose is correct. However, if most high blood glucose levels are followed by hypoglycemic levels, then the supplemental dose is too high. Conversely, if most high levels are followed by another high level, then the supplemental dose is too low. The patient should be advised to decrease or increase the sensitivity factor in the supplemental formula as needed to achieve the desired change in the blood glucose level. (Refer to Chapter 6, *Bolus and Supplemental Insulin*, for instructions.)

To adjust premeal bolus doses, one focuses on the pattern of blood glucose levels before lunch, dinner, and bedtime. If the blood glucose levels at the same time of day (e.g., before dinner) are high **two days** in a row, then this indicates a need to increase the preceding premeal (e.g., before lunch) bolus by one unit (or 10 percent). Conversely, a **single** low blood glucose indicates the need to decrease the preceding premeal bolus by one unit. Changing this bolus dose the very next day will prevent a recurrence of hypoglycemia and thereby protect against the establishment of reduced hypoglycemic awareness (4).

Adjustment of overnight basal rates is guided by pattern analysis of the 3 AM and prebreakfast levels, taking into account the preceding level. For example, if the 3 AM blood glucose is high for two days in a row, with a normal bedtime blood glucose, the primary basal rate (profile #1) is increased by 0.1 unit per hour. If the 3 AM blood glucose is low even once, the primary basal rate is lowered by 0.1 unit per hour. Similar pattern analysis and basal rate adjustment for the 3 AM to 7 AM "window" is done using the prebreakfast blood glucose levels. If there is marked fluctuation in the daytime or evening blood glucose levels, the basal rate during these time periods should be tested and adjusted accordingly. Protocols for testing and adjusting basal rates are described in detail in Chapter 5, *Establishing & Verifying Basal Insulin Rates*.

We check the data from the pump's memory (the last seven boluses and the last week's daily totals) during a visit to verify recordkeeping.

Guidelines for Adjusting Premeal Bolus And Overnight Basal Insulin Doses Based on Blood Glucose Pattern Analysis*

Blood Glucose Level	If HIGH 2 days in a row, take the following action	If LOW once, take the following action:
3 AM	**Increase** basal rate profile #1 from midnight-3 AM by 0.1 U/h.	**Decrease** basal rate profile #1 from midnight-3 AM by 0.1 U/h.
Prebreakfast	**Increase** dawn basal (profile #2) from 3-9 AM by 0.1 U/h.	**Decrease** dawn basal (profile #2) from 3-9 AM by 0.1 U/h.
Prelunch	**Increase** prebreakfast bolus by 1 unit OR skip breakfast and test BG at 9 and 11 AM to determine if dawn basal should be continued longer.**	**Decrease** prebreakfast bolus by 1 unit OR skip breakfast and test BG at 9 and 11 AM to determine if dawn basal should be stopped earlier.**
Presupper	**Increase** prelunch bolus by 1 unit.	**Decrease** prelunch bolus by 1 unit.
Bedtime	**Increase** presupper bolus by 1 unit.	**Decrease** presupper bolus by 1 unit.

* Generally, adjustment of premeal bolus doses corrects out-of-range blood glucose values in the daytime and evening hours. If not, the basal rate during the affected time period should be tested and adjusted according to the protocol in Chapter 5.

** Never start basal testing unless blood glucose is in target range. See Chapter 5.

SUMMARY

Regular blood glucose monitoring, recordkeeping and pattern analysis help ensure the safety and effectiveness of pump-based intensive insulin therapy. The recordkeeping and pattern analysis systems described here have been used in our clinical practice for over ten years and have assisted our pump users in improving glycemic control while reducing rates of both severe hypoglycemia and diabetic ketoacidosis (3). Other useful systems of recordkeeping and analysis exist; the key is to implement a logical, comprehensive system that pump users and the diabetes team can use as a basis for effective communication and therapeutic management.

The key is to implement a logical, comprehensive system that pump users and the diabetes team can use as a basis for effective communication and therapeutic management.

CASE STUDIES IN PATTERN ANALYSIS

Case Study #1: Overnight Basal Rate

Steve F., a 39-year old hospital manager, has been using an insulin pump for three months. His control has improved and he is seeing less variation in his blood glucose using one basal rate (0.8 U/h). His bolus doses are 6 units before each of three meals of equal carbohydrate content, and his supplemental doses are based on the formula (BG-100)/40. Steve's target blood glucose range is 70 to 150 mg/dL.

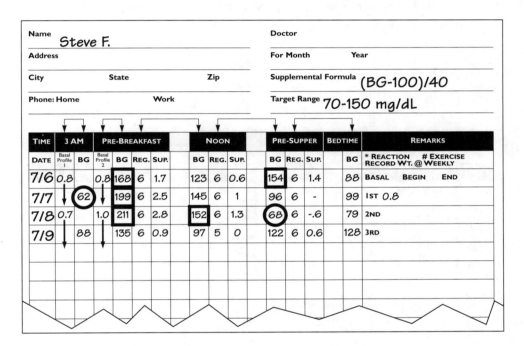

Name					Doctor			
Steve F.								

Address

Doctor

For Month   Year

City   State   Zip

Supplemental Formula (BG-100)/40

Phone: Home   Work

Target Range 70-150 mg/dL

TIME	3 AM		PRE-BREAKFAST				NOON			PRE-SUPPER			BEDTIME	REMARKS
DATE	Basal Profile 1	BG	Basal Profile 2	BG	REG.	SUP.	BG	REG.	SUP.	BG	REG.	SUP.	BG	* REACTION # EXERCISE RECORD WT. @ WEEKLY
7/6	0.8		0.8	168	6	1.7		123	6	0.6	154	6	1.4	88	BASAL BEGIN END
7/7		62		199	6	2.5		145	6	1	96	6	-	99	1ST 0.8
7/8	0.7		1.0	211	6	2.8		152	6	1.3	68	6	-.6	79	2ND
7/9		88		135	6	0.9		97	5	0	122	6	0.6	128	3RD

The following is Steve's blood glucose record for the past four days:

Comparison of daily patterns, facilitated by the one-page recordkeeping format, shows that Steve's 3 AM blood glucose levels are in the normal to low range, while his morning values have risen considerably.

To correct this pattern, we would advise Steve to reduce his basal rate from midnight to 3 AM by 0.1 unit per hour, to 0.7 unit per hour. As he is seeing a >30 mg/dL rise from 3AM until prebreakfast, he should implement a second basal rate of 1.0 unit per hour starting at 3 AM and continuing to 9 AM on 7/8. Then from 9 AM until midnight his basal rate should revert back to 0.8 unit per hour.

Once Steve's 3 AM and prebreakfast blood glucose levels are within target, he should test the dawn and morning basal rate "windows" by skipping breakfast and testing blood glucose levels every two hours. This will help him both to verify the accuracy of the basal rates and to know when to change from the dawn basal rate to the lower, daytime rate.

Case Study #2: Bolus Dosing

John F., who has a history of reduced hypoglycemic awareness, has been on an insulin pump for three weeks. He is consuming three equal carbohydrate meals, with no snacks. John's premeal bolus dose is 7 units and his basal rate is 0.9 unit per hour. Because of his reduced hypoglycemic awareness, John's target blood glucose range is 80 to 160 mg/dL and his supplemental insulin is calculated from the formula (BG-120)/35.

Shown below is a four-day section of John's flow sheet. It is apparent from the flow sheet that John is experiencing persistently elevated presupper blood glucose levels:

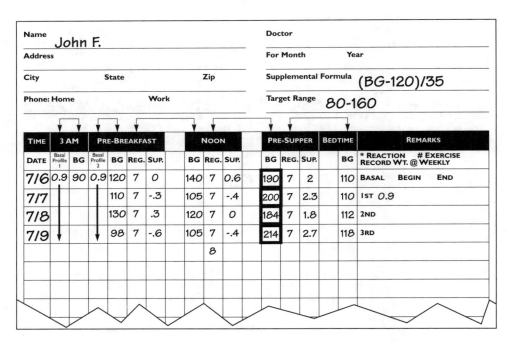

John's supplemental dose seems to be correct, as each high predinner blood glucose is followed by a bedtime blood glucose level in the normal range. He should increase his prelunch bolus by 1 unit, to 8 units, to correct the pattern of high predinner blood glucose levels.

Case Study #3: Supplemental Insulin

Susan H. is a 25-year old woman who has been on an insulin pump for one year. Recently, she has been seeing a pattern of low bedtime blood glucose levels. Susan has been careful to calculate her predinner boluses according to her usual carbohydrate to insulin ratio, which is 15/1, and to calculate her supplemental insulin boluses using her usual sensitivity factor of 45, i.e., (BG-100)/45. Her blood glucose log for the past four days appears below:

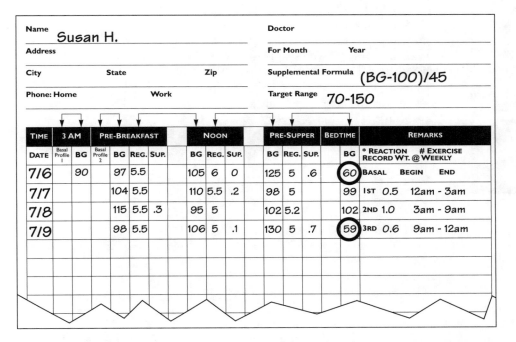

Name	Susan H.											Doctor			

Name: Susan H.
Doctor:
Address:
For Month: Year:
City: State: Zip:
Supplemental Formula: (BG-100)/45
Phone: Home   Work
Target Range: 70-150

TIME	3 AM		PRE-BREAKFAST				NOON			PRE-SUPPER			BEDTIME	REMARKS
DATE	Basal Profile 1	BG	Basal Profile 2	BG	REG.	SUP.	BG	REG.	SUP.	BG	REG.	SUP.	BG	* REACTION # EXERCISE RECORD WT. @ WEEKLY
7/6		90		97	5.5		105	6	0	125	5	.6	(60)	BASAL BEGIN END
7/7				104	5.5		110	5.5	.2	98	5		99	1ST 0.5 12am - 3am
7/8				115	5.5	.3	95	5		102	5.2		102	2ND 1.0 3am - 9am
7/9				98	5.5		106	5	.1	130	5	.7	(59)	3RD 0.6 9am - 12am

Susan's levels are low at bedtime on the days she takes predinner supplemental insulin, and within target on the days she uses no supplement. This may indicate that she is more sensitive to insulin later in the day. She should raise her sensitivity factor by 10 points at dinner to see if this brings the bedtime levels back into the target range. Susan will now begin to calculate her predinner supplement using the formula (BG-100)/55, but continue to use her preexisting supplemental formula to calculate prebreakfast and prelunch supplements.

Supplemental doses are recorded separately from premeal boluses to permit analysis of their effect.

REFERENCES

1. American Diabetes Association. Self-monitoring of blood glucose. *Diabetes Care* 1993;18(Suppl 1):47-52.

2. Farkas-Hirsch R, Hirsch IB. Continuous subcutaneous insulin infusion: a review of the past and its implementation for the future. *Diabetes Spectrum* 1994;7:80-84.

3. Bode B, Steed D, Davidson P. Long-term pump use and SMBG in 205 patients. *Diabetes* 1994;43(Suppl 1):220A.

4. Cryer PE. Hypoglycemia begets hypoglycemia in IDDM. *Diabetes* 1993; 42:1691-1693.

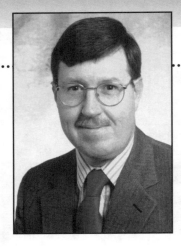

WILLIAM E. DUDLEY II, MD, CDE

Dr. Dudley is a practicing endocrinologist and Medical Director of the Seacoast Diabetes Institute in Dover, N.H. Past President of the New Hampshire Affiliate of the American Diabetes Association and cofounder of Camp Carefree, a summer camp for children with diabetes, Dr. Dudley is also a member of the American College of Clinical Endocrinologists and the American Association of Diabetes Educators.

MARY JO DUDLEY, RN, BSN, CDE

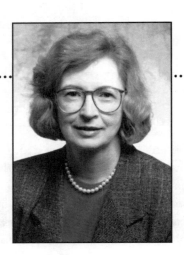

Mary Jo Dudley is Program Director of the Seacoast Diabetes Institute and was the 1994 recipient of the McBean-Little Award as the outstanding Diabetes Educator in New Hampshire. Past president of the New Hampshire Chapter of Diabetes Educators, Ms. Dudley is a MiniMed Certified Pump Trainer and a frequent lecturer in New England. She writes diabetes education literature for both consumer and professional audiences.

Everyday Management

Pumps go wherever people go, which might include sky-diving, climbing Mount Everest, spelunking, playing college rugby, visiting the White House, and attending cheerleading competitions. Most pump users are thus keenly interested in learning how their day-to-day activities—including the unusual or delicate ones—will be affected by switching from injection therapy to continuous subcutaneous insulin infusion (CSII). Common questions include: "Will people notice I'm wearing a pump?" "Will I still be able to swim?... take a shower? ... have sex with my partner?... travel to Asia next year?... pass through airport security?... use my new hot tub?... sleep in the nude?... go horseback riding?"

Such questions about everyday life with the pump often need to be addressed first, before the prospective pump user receives instruction in the details of pump operation (1). This chapter provides some specific guidelines to help pump users incorporate CSII therapy into the activities of their daily lives. For details on sports and exercise with the pump, refer to Chapter 10, *Exercise & the Pump*.

SHOWERING AND BATHING

The insulin pump is an electromechanical instrument and might be damaged by water; therefore, care must be taken to prevent the electronic components from getting wet. Pump casings give some measure of protection, but precautions are still needed to protect the pump when bathing or showering.

There are several methods for protecting the pump or disconnecting from the pump when bathing or showering:

IN THIS CHAPTER

Swimming & Showering

Sleeping

Sexual Intimacy

Travel

Illness

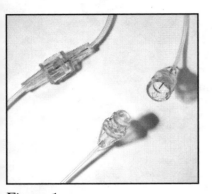

Figure 1

Quick Release™ infusion set connector.

- The Quick Release™* is an infusion set option which allows for easy temporary disconnection from the pump. The QR connector, located several inches from the infusion site, allows the user to temporarily disconnect from the pump without having to change the infusion set. This is particularly helpful while bathing or showering, drying off, and dressing.
- The SportGuard™* is a protective case designed to be used during all types of physical activities. It completely protects the pump from water or physical damage and can be used during bathing or showering with excellent results.
- The ShowerPak™* is a specially designed plastic bag that holds the pump during showering. It can hang from the shower head or faucet handle or around the pump user's neck.
- The pump can be placed on the side of the tub during a bath. However, it is recommended that the Quick Release be used or the pump be placed in the SportGuard to prevent damage in the event that it accidentally falls into the tub.

Available from MiniMed Technologies, Sylmar, CA

HOT TUBS, SAUNAS AND SUNBATHING

While using either a hot tub or sauna, the pump user can temporarily disconnect from the pump. Use of the Quick Release is recommended for this purpose. If the pump user chooses not to disconnect the pump, he or she should be aware that the high temperature may affect insulin potency.

When sunbathing, the pump user should protect the pump and insulin from direct sunlight by placing a towel over it. The pump can be removed temporarily, for periods up to one hour (2). Removal for longer than one hour is not recommended unless the pump user has taken a bolus of insulin or insulin by injection.

If the tape holding the infusion set becomes loose (from water jet pressure or perspiration), the infusion cannula may become dislodged. Loose tape, therefore, is a sign that the entire infusion set should be changed immediately.

During and after periods of pump removal or exposure to heat, blood glucose levels should be checked frequently. Because heat increases insulin absorption, there is an increased risk of developing hypoglycemia (3,4). Hyperglycemia can occur when the insulin in the infusion set has been affected adversely by the heat. Pump users should therefore change the reservoir and infusion set whenever an unexplained high blood glucose occurs. This is especially important when activities that occurred during pump removal may have caused the infusion set to become dislodged.

SPECIAL OCCASIONS

For special occasions such as proms, weddings or just a night out, the pump user may want to hide the pump or may need to find a new location for it if the outfit is not conducive to wearing it in the usual spot. Women learn to be creative in the way they wear their pump (5), placing it in their bra, panty hose (support hose) or on a garter. Men can place the pump in the pocket of their pants, on a belt or in a passport holder worn under their clothes. The Sock-it-Away, a leg pouch designed to be worn under the pants leg, is particularly useful for men or for women wearing long skirts or pants.

SLEEPING

Bedtime activities are often the most anxiety-producing for a new pump user. He or she may fear that the pump will interfere with regular sleep habits or that the infusion set will become disconnected or dislodged during sleep. With the 42-inch tubing available on all types of MiniMed infusion sets, the pump can be placed beneath the pillow or on the bedside stand and still accommodate the most restless sleeper with ease. This extended length tubing provides the necessary freedom for those who sleep in the nude. For those who prefer pajamas or nightgowns, the pump can be placed in a pocket, allowing full movement while sleeping. Stomach sleepers report that they encounter no discomfort while sleeping using either the Sof-set™ or a bent needle.

SEXUAL INTIMACY

Most prospective pump users are concerned about what to do with the pump during sexual activity, but may not feel comfortable asking about it. The subject should be brought up by the health care provider so that fears can by allayed. Most concerns can be dispelled if partners discuss them openly. According to C. Sannar in a survey of 100 pump users at Mason Clinic, couples usually find that wearing the pump during sexual activity does not interfere with sexual intimacy (6).

Tubing occasionally gets pulled on during sexual activity. In fact, many couples joke about tangles with the infusion set. This is not harmful, although the tape and infusion set should be checked carefully after sexual activity to be sure the system is still intact. If the tubing does become detached during sexual activity, the pump should be set aside and replaced afterwards. Partners should be assured that nothing terrible (the pump user won't bleed to death!) will happen if the tubing becomes detached.

The Quick Release can be used to disconnect during periods of intimacy. If the time off the pump will be greater than one hour, insulin replacement will be needed. The pump user should be cautioned against falling asleep before the pump is replaced.

Options for Wearing the Pump

- *Belt clip*
- *Leather cases*
- *Pockets of pants, skirts, shirts or pajamas*
- *Inside support panty hose*

  Bra pouch
- *Inside tennis panties*
- *Sock-it-Away leg pouch*
- *Garter belts*

Insulin Pump Identification Card

ATTENTION: A medical device containing metal is being worn by the bearer of this card. This device cannot be removed.

"I have insulin-dependent diabetes mellitus and am wearing an insulin pump which delivers insulin continuously into the subcutaneous tissue to control my diabetes."

DO NOT REMOVE
THIS PUMP.

Name
_____

Address
_____

_____

City, State
_____

Zip
_____

Additional Notes on Pump Disconnection

- The pump should be removed whenever an x-ray, CAT scan or MRI is to take place. By using an infusion set with the Quick Release disconnect feature, the pump user can easily reconnect the pump after the procedure.

- The convenient disconnect feature of the Quick Release might make it easier to misplace the pump in a purse, locker room or dressing room. Therefore, a pump user should be advised to check with his or her homeowners insurance policy regarding coverage of the pump if it is lost or stolen.

TRAVEL

An insulin pump makes traveling across time zones easier for a person with diabetes. The pump user will want to carry a card or letter explaining the necessity of carrying diabetes supplies and equipment, especially when traveling across international borders. The pump user should also carry extra diabetes and pump supplies (insulin, additional infusion sets and reservoirs, insulin syringes, and blood glucose testing supplies) as well as snacks in his or her CARRY ON luggage. Insulin should not be left in checked luggage as it may freeze or go to another destination.

Travel Letter Example

(Name, address, and phone number
of doctor's office or hospital
should be placed here)

To Whom It May Concern:

_____ is a patient in this office being treated for insulin-requiring diabetes mellitus. He/she is currently using an insulin pump and does blood sugar monitoring by finger stick. Hypoglycemic reactions (low blood sugars) are always a possibility, requiring treatment with glucose tablets or acceptable substitutes. Therefore, it is essential that he/she have in his/her possession at all times insulin, insulin syringes and the equipment to test his/her blood sugar levels. It is also essential that he/she wear the insulin pump at all times, as it is continuously supplying the drug, insulin, which is required for the patient's survival.

If you have any questions, please contact this office.

Yours truly,

(MD's signature)

International travelers should be advised to carry antidiarrhea and antinausea medications, conventional insulin supplies (and dosage schedule), ketone test strips and glucagon. They need to perform more frequent blood glucose tests and to be extra cautious regarding food and beverage choices and daily self-care routines.

When traveling across time zones, the clock in the pump must be readjusted. This will compensate for any change in the duration of basal profiles due to gain or loss of hours.

Pump users report varying degrees of success in traveling through airport metal detectors without causing the alarm to be activated. The sensitivity of these alarms varies from airport to airport and from day to day, but insulin pumps should trigger them no more frequently than the metal on a felt tip pen. One pump user who travels extensively in the US, Europe and Asia reports triggering the alarm only once out of 25 recent trips. When the airport security person noticed the pump while scanning her, she explained that it was an insulin pump, and the security person accepted this explanation. European airport security personnel tend to be familiar with insulin pumps, as CSII is common in Europe. Language barriers can, however, present occasional problems.

When dealing with airport security systems:
- Don't point out the pump beforehand.
- If the alarm goes off, don't point out the pump, as the alarm may have been triggered by a belt or an earring.
- Don't look overly anxious, as this causes the security guards to pay more attention.
- Carry a card or letter from your physician in case further explanation is needed.

During extended travel, the pump user may want to have the name of an endocrinologist in the area he or she will be visiting. The American Diabetes Association can provide the names of qualified professionals in different travel destinations. The phone number for the American Diabetes Association is: (800)ADA-DISC (inside the US); (703)549-1500 (outside the US). MiniMed has offices worldwide and can also assist in locating a local endocrinologist. To call MiniMed from outside the US, dial (818)362-5958.

ILLNESS

An acute illness such as flu, diarrhea, bronchitis, or even the common cold, can be dangerous to any person with diabetes. Prompt and decisive action, however, can almost always prevent severe problems for a pump user. Because diabetic

When dealing with airport security systems: If the alarm goes off, don't point out the pump, as the alarm may have been triggered by a belt or an earring. Carry a card or letter from your physician in case further explanation is needed.

ketoacidosis (DKA) is a possible risk with CSII, pump users should be prepared to act quickly if an illness should interrupt their blood glucose control (see Chapter 11, *DKA Prevention*).

The sample sick day rules outlined here are effective most of the time in controlling out-of-range blood glucose values and in clearing ketones from the blood and urine. The rules are similar to those provided by most institutions (7). Pump users should be instructed to follow such guidelines carefully and completely whenever illness occurs and to call the health care team if blood glucose remains elevated, ketones do not resolve, or vomiting occurs.

SICK DAY RULES FOR PUMP USERS

When an illness occurs:

1. Always take your insulin. NEVER omit your basal insulin, even if you are unable to eat. Do not remove your pump, unless you are taking adequate amounts of insulin via injections.

2. Begin testing blood glucose and urine ketones as soon as illness starts and continue to test every 2 to 4 hours, 24 hours a day. Keep an accurate record of the test results.

3. If the blood glucose is higher than 200 mg/dL, discontinue meals and push fluids (sugar-free) to clear ketones. Take supplemental doses of insulin, calculated according to your supplemental formula, as follows:
   - If ketones are not present, take supplemental insulin every 4 hours until the blood glucose level falls below 200 mg/dL.
   - If ketones are present, take supplemental insulin every 2 hours until the blood glucose has returned to near-target levels and ketones are improving.

4. When the blood glucose returns to near-target, carbohydrates need to be taken to clear the ketones. Take an appropriate presnack bolus and drink or eat sugar-containing clear fluids such as regular soda, Jell-O, or popsicles.

5. Plan ahead for sick days. Have a Sick Day Kit readily available. It should contain the following supplies:
   - Telephone number of doctor and/or diabetes educator.
   - Sugar-containing clear fluids (apple juice, regular cola, popsicles, gelatin) to replace solid food.
   - Syringes and extra vials of insulin to combat very high blood glucose levels and urine ketones.
   - Glucagon kit in case of severe hypoglycemia
   - Extra supplies for urine ketone testing and increased blood glucose monitoring.
   - Thermometer

- Medication for fever (such as Tylenol)
- Sugar-free cough drops or syrup
- An antidiarrheal such as Immodium
- An antinausea agent such as Compazine suppositories

6. Call your doctor if you have any of the following DANGER SIGNALS:
   - Persistent nausea
   - Vomiting more than once in 4 to 6 hours
   - Moderate or large urine ketones
   - You cannot get blood glucose or ketones down after 2 supplemental insulin doses
   - When in doubt about anything CALL your health care provider!

RETURNING TO MULTIPLE DAILY INJECTIONS

In the event that the pump user needs to temporarily discontinue pump use, he or she needs to know how to return to a regimen of multiple daily injections (MDI). Because pump users become so accustomed to the pump, they are often reluctant even to discuss returning to conventional insulin injections. However, it is imperative that the health care provider explain and provide a conventional insulin regimen using multiple daily injections as an alternative to CSII. Having an injection protocol on hand will ensure that the pump user is prepared for unexpected problems and will save the doctor or nurse from receiving phone calls in the middle of the night.

INFUSION SITE PROBLEMS AND SOLUTIONS

Proper care of the infusion set and site are essential to successful pump therapy and personal comfort. The diabetes health care provider needs to be well informed about infusion site care in order to help the pump user prevent site-related problems and solve any that may occur.

Skin Irritation

Skin irritation may be caused by sensitivity to the tape being used, or by friction from the needle or plastic parts of the infusion set. Skin irritation also may be the first sign of an infection. The infusion site should therefore be checked or changed at the first sign of irritation or discomfort. Taking action immediately will keep little problems from turning into more serious problems.

If irritation appears wherever the tape touches the skin, the pump user may be sensitive to the tape's adhesive or material. Switching to another brand of tape is often the simplest way to solve this problem, as different tapes use different materials and adhesives. Removing tape adhesive from the skin with a product made for this purpose (Unisolve, Smith and Nephew United) may ease irrita-

Guidelines for Switching To Multiple Daily Injections

1. If pump use is to be suspended for fewer than 3 to 4 days, continue using regular insulin on a schedule of 5 injections per day.

2. Check blood glucose every 4 to 5 hours.

3. Each premeal injection should include the following:
   a. Premeal bolus based on usual carbohydrate/insulin ratio.
   b. 3 hours of the usual basal dose
   c. Supplemental insulin is added or subtracted based on the premeal blood glucose level according to the person's usual supplemental formula.

4. At bedtime, inject 3 hours of the usual basal dose plus any necessary supplemental insulin.

5. In the middle of the sleep period, inject 3 hours of the usual basal dose plus any necessary supplemental insulin.

6. If pump use will be discontinued for more than 3 or 4 days, regular insulin should be taken before meals according to the above schedule, and the usual basal dose for the overnight period may be taken as NPH at bedtime.

If perspiration is a problem, try applying antiperspirant or Skin Tac "H" around the insertion site, and under the area that will be covered by tape or dressing.

tion caused by the adhesive. Mineral, olive or baby oil can also be used to remove tape residue from the skin. The oil can either be washed off with soap and water or wiped off with alcohol.

Irritation from the plastic parts of the infusion set may be prevented by first putting a layer of tape or dressing against the skin, and then inserting the infusion set through this. Once the set is in place, it should be secured with a second layer of tape.

Metal sensitivity is another possible cause of irritation. If irritation occurs in areas that come in contact with a metal needle, use of the Sof-set™ may alleviate the problem.

Tape Adhesion Problems

If the tape or Sof-set dressing is not sticking properly, holding the hand over the tape for one to two minutes after application will warm the tape and may improve adhesion. This technique can be used with any tape or dressing. Switching tape brands also may solve problems with poor adhesion.

One of the most common causes of poor sticking is perspiration. This is a particular challenge for people who are physically active or live in hot climates. If perspiration is a problem, try applying antiperspirant or Skin Tac "H" (see Skin Barriers) around the insertion site, and under the area that will be covered by tape or dressing. Avoid the actual insertion site to prevent antiperspirant being carried into the skin when the needle or cannula is inserted. Make sure the antiperspirant has dried completely before proceeding.

If perspiration has moistened the tape or dressing holding a metal needle infusion set in place, it is possible to remove the tape without disturbing the needle. If this can be done successfully, dry the area thoroughly and retape. However, always replace the Sof-set if the dressing begins to peel. A loose dressing may allow the cannula to become dislodged.

Insulin Absorption Problems

Hyperglycemia can be a sign that an infusion site has ceased to absorb insulin properly. Absorption problems can be caused by hypertrophy (tissue build-up) or infection at the infusion site, or by a bent Sof-set catheter.

Hypertrophy can result from injecting insulin repeatedly into the same site or from leaving the infusion set in too long. Skin or underlying tissue that feels hard, solid, or tough is a sign of hypertrophy. If this occurs, the pump user should avoid infusing into the affected area, including one inch around it, for at least one month to give the damaged area time to heal. If insulin is injected into damaged areas before the tissue has returned to normal, poor or unpredictable insulin absorption may result, and the tissue damage may worsen.

TAPES AND DRESSINGS

Polyskin (Kendall —available from MiniMed). A transparent dressing compatible with most skin types, Polyskin is intended for people with allergies and sensitivities. It adheres well when exposed to moisture and comes in a convenient 2" x 2.7" size that is perfect for covering the infusion set. If used with the Sof-set, the tape will be more comfortable if a hole is cut in the center. This can be done by folding the tape in fourths and cutting off the folded corner to accommodate the Sof-set.

Tegaderm or TegadermHP (3M) and **IV 3000** (Smith and Nephew United) are both transparent dressings. **Compeed** (Bruder Medical Products Division) is a dressing that adheres well when wet.

Hypafix (Smith and Nephew United) is a white (non-transparent) roll tape with very good adhesive. **HyTape** (Hy Pink Surgical), a pink fabric roll tape, is also reported to demonstrate good adherence. **Transpore** (3M) and **Dermicell** (Johnson and Johnson) are clear roll tapes that stick well and are used by many pump users to secure safety loops.

Other types include silk tape, which sticks extremely well and comes off fairly easily when pulled, and paper tape, used by people who have extremely sensitive skin. Paper tape, however, does not adhere as well as other products.

Skin Barriers

Skin preparations that place a barrier between the skin and the tape's adhesive help prevent irritation and sensitivity problems. These products also help tape stick better. Be sure that the infusion site dries thoroughly after applying these products, before trying to apply a tape or dressing. **SkinPrep** (United, Division of Howmedica) is a protective dressing for sensitive skin which is wiped on before placing tape onto the skin. **Skin Tac "H"** (Mason Labs, Inc.) is a liquid adhesive which is brushed on the skin before applying tape to help the tape stick better.

SUMMARY

With a little ingenuity and a lot of common sense, the pump user can incorporate the insulin pump into day-to-day routines, as well as travel, sports, and unusual activities. Pump accessories such as the Quick Release, SportGuard, ShowerPak, and Sock-it-Away facilitate pump protection and concealment and simplify temporary disconnection, when needed. Traveling with a pump requires several special precautions, including more frequent blood glucose monitoring and the carrying of extra supplies and a medical identification letter or card. All pump users should know the protocol for temporarily returning to multiple daily injections in the event that this becomes necessary. Sick day guidelines for pump users do not differ greatly from those for people on conventional injection therapy, and should be follow scrupulously, under the supervision of the diabetes care team. Solutions to some common infusion site problems are presented; complete infusion site care information can be found in Chapter 4, *Initiating Pump Therapy*.

REFERENCES

1. Farkas-Hirsch R, Levandoski L. Implementation of continuous subcutaneous insulin infusion therapy: an overview. *Diabetes Educ* 1988;14:401-406.

2. Strowig SM. Initiation and management of insulin pump therapy. *Diabetes Educ* 1993;19:50-59.

3. Koivisto VA. Sauna-induced acceleration in insulin absorption from subcutaneous injection site. *Br Med J* 1980;280:1411-1413.

4. Koivisto VA, Fortney S, Hendler R, Felig P. A rise in ambient temperature augments insulin absorption in diabetic patients. *Metabolism* 1981;30:402-405.

5. Farkas-Hirsch R, Hirsch IB. Continuous subcutaneous insulin infusion: A review of the past and its implementation for the future. *Diabetes Spectrum* 1994;7:80-84.

6. Sannar C. Personal communication. Virginia Mason Clinic, Seattle, WA, 1986.

7. Brackenridge BP, D'Almeida B, Fredrickson, LP, Swenson K. About sick days. In: *The Pump Trainer Manual*. Sylmar, CA: MiniMed Technologies; 1994;55.

8. Mecklenburg RS, Benson EA, Benson JW, Fredlund PN, Guinn T, Metz RJ, Nielsen, RL, Sannar CA. Acute complications associated with insulin infusion pump therapy. Report of experience with 161 patients. *JAMA* 1984;252:3265-3269.

9. Skyler, JS. Continuous subcutaneous insulin infusion (CSII) with external devices: current status. In: Ensminger WD, Selam JL, eds. *Update in Drug Delivery Systems*. Mount Kisco, NY: Futura; 1989;163-183.

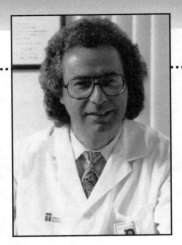

BERNARD ZINMAN, MDCM, FRCPC, FACP

Dr. Zinman is Professor of Medicine and Director of the Banting and Best Diabetes Centre at the University of Toronto, and Head of the Division of Endocrinology and Metabolism at the Mount Sinai and Toronto Hospitals. He was principal investigator for the University of Toronto center of the DCCT and served as Chair of the Treatment Committee for this study. Dr. Zinman's major research interests are in the prevention of the long-term complications of diabetes, the assessment of insulin action and beta cell function in various states of abnormal nutrition, the evaluation of the metabolic responses to exercise, and the investigation of the epidemiology of diabetes and related disorders in native North Americans.

EXERCISE & THE PUMP

10

Exercise is important for all people with diabetes; however, exercise recommendations for individuals with non-insulin dependent diabetes (NIDDM) differ from those for people with insulin-dependent diabetes (IDDM). In people with NIDDM, exercise is an important part of daily management. Even modest degrees of exercise can improve metabolic control by enhancing insulin sensitivity, promoting weight loss and helping to maintain weight reduction. In people with IDDM, exercise in and of itself has not been shown to have a beneficial effect on long-term glycemic control (1,2); however, its many positive non-glycemic effects can enhance both health and quality of life. Exercise improves cardiovascular fitness, lowers blood pressure, improves the lipid profile by increasing HDL cholesterol and lowering LDL cholesterol, and contributes to an improved sense of well-being (3).

Exercise may be a leisure activity, occurring infrequently and spontaneously; competitive, occurring on a regular basis, two to three times per week; or high-intensity training, as exemplified by amateur and professional athletes. People with IDDM who enjoy exercise and active sports need to learn how to adjust their diet and/or insulin regimen to allow safe participation in their favorite activities. This chapter focuses on the therapeutic modifications required for exercise participation by persons using continuous subcutaneous insulin infusion (CSII).

IN THIS CHAPTER

Physiologic Responses

Modifying Treatment

Case Studies

Water Sports

Contact Sports

PHYSIOLOGIC RESPONSES TO EXERCISE

To better understand the rationale for adjusting the treatment regimen in response to exercise, it is useful to review the normal hormonal and metabolic responses to exercise. Several important variables determine a person's metabolic response to exercise, including his or her fitness level, metabolic state (fasting or postprandial) at the start of exercise, and the intensity and duration of the exercise. Irrespective of the type of exercise, the principal metabolic goal is to provide energy substrate to the contracting muscle to allow the performance of meaningful work (4,5).

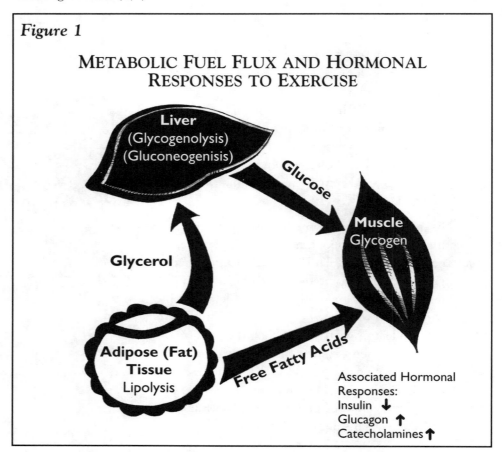

Figure 1

METABOLIC FUEL FLUX AND HORMONAL RESPONSES TO EXERCISE

Muscle glycogen serves as the first readily available energy source, particularly in the early phases of strenuous exercise. As exercise continues, circulating fuels, primarily glucose, take on a more prominent role. Glucose is mobilized from the liver by the process of glycogenolysis (the breakdown of hepatic glycogen) and gluconeogenesis (the formation of glucose from 3-carbon precursors). Under most circumstances the increase in muscle glucose utilization is precisely and synchronously matched by changes in hepatic glucose production. As a consequence, circulating glucose levels remain remarkably constant and the brain, which has an obligate need for glucose, has an adequate substrate supply.

Finally, with prolonged exercise, adipose tissue stores become important in providing a sustained source of energy for contracting muscle. Free fatty acids are mobilized from adipose tissue by the process of lipolysis (the breakdown of triglyceride to three free fatty acids and glycerol) and are bound to circulating albumin for transport to the muscle. In addition the glycerol released from adipose tissue can serve as a gluconeogenic substrate for the liver. The sequence of these events, although similar in all individuals, will vary depending on an individual's fitness and the intensity and duration of exercise.

These complex metabolic responses, illustrated in Figure 1, are controlled by the cardiovascular system, the central nervous system and, most importantly in the context of IDDM, the endocrine system. Insulin and its counterregulatory hormones (glucagon, catecholamines) play pivotal roles in controlling metabolic fuel flux in response to exercise. Insulin is a potent inhibitor of the mobilization of both glucose from the liver and free fatty acids from adipose tissue; thus basal insulin levels normally decrease by approximately 50 percent with exercise (6,7). This lowered basal level of insulin is required for normal fuel flux during exercise. (An absolute deficiency of insulin will result in impaired glucose uptake, hyperglycemia and ketosis.) Glucagon stimulates hepatic glucose production, while catecholamines enhance adipose tissue lipolysis.

MODIFYING THE DIABETES TREATMENT REGIMEN IN ANTICIPATION OF EXERCISE

To compensate for exercise and to maintain adequate glycemic control, the diabetes treatment regimen can be modified by increasing caloric intake, adjusting the insulin dose, or both. The latter approach is particularly advantageous if one is concerned about weight gain, and can best be utilized by individuals on intensive treatment regimens, who have multiple opportunities to adjust the insulin dosage throughout the day. A major advantage of CSII is the degree of flexibility it permits in insulin dose adjustment for exercise.

Although general guidelines can be provided with respect to basal and premeal bolus insulin changes for exercise, it must be recognized that individual responses vary considerably. Thus, self-monitoring of blood glucose (SMBG) is an essential component of any exercise insulin adjustment strategy and helps establish the glycemic response to a particular activity. This information is also invaluable in evaluating the response to modification in insulin therapy. As an example, it has been clearly demonstrated that with high-intensity, strenuous exercise of short duration, hyperglycemia, rather than hypoglycemia, commonly occurs (8). In this case, insulin dose adjustment may not be required for the exercise, but is essential in the postexercise period.

In the following guidelines we have adhered to the principle that changes should be kept simple, be consistent with the known physiologic responses to

A major advantage of CSII is the degree of flexibility it permits in insulin dose adjustment for exercise.

Basal rate adjustments are the most appropriate insulin delivery change when exercise is being performed before breakfast or when four to six hours have passed since the last meal bolus.

exercise, and serve as a starting point for further insulin dose adjustment based on SMBG information. Depending on the type of exercise, the pump user may benefit from wearing the pump during exercise or by removing it temporarily. Both pump-on and pump-off options are therefore presented. In addition to these specific recommendations, there are several important general principles that are applicable to any individual with IDDM who would like to initiate an exercise program. These are summarized in Table I.

Table I

GUIDELINES FOR EXERCISE IN IDDM

I.   **Assess Clinical Status**
  - Assess metabolic status
  - Evaluate cardiovascular health
  - Document complication status

II. **Establish Appropriate Exercise Program**
  - Intensity
  - Duration
  - Frequency

III. **Educate Participant Regarding:**
  - Importance of self-monitoring of blood glucose
  - Recognition of immediate and delayed hypoglycemia
  - Risk of ketosis
  - Insulin dose adjustment strategies
  - Importance of fluid replacement
  - Need for carbohydrate supplementation
  - Prevention of injury (e.g. stretching, footwear, etc.)

PUMP-ON STRATEGIES

It is preferable to maintain insulin infusion during exercise in order to benefit fully from the unique insulin dose adjustment characteristics of CSII. Wearing the pump permits systematic and logical modification of basal and bolus insulin.

Basal Insulin Modification

Basal rate adjustments are the most appropriate insulin delivery change when exercise is being performed before breakfast or when four to six hours have passed since the last meal bolus. The latter situation is often the case when participating in late afternoon workouts or sports events. Changes in the infusion rate are determined by the duration and intensity of the exercise activity and the individual's level of conditioning. A person who is well-conditioned may require only small, if any, changes in the basal rate with exercise. Selecting the appropriate Temporary Basal insulin infusion rate when exercise is initiated before breakfast can result in remarkably stable glycemic control without the need to consume extra calories.

A useful starting point is to decrease the basal rate to half the usual infusion rate for the duration of the activity. As an example, the usual basal infusion rate may be 1.2 units per hour. When exercise is initiated the rate is reduced to 0.6 unit per hour (temporary basal) for the duration of the exercise, which may be 45 minutes of jogging, or 60 minutes of tennis or other moderate activity. When the activity is finished, the usual basal rate is reinstituted. Some individuals prefer to reduce the basal rate 30 to 60 minutes before starting exercise. This allows the insulin level to drop before exercise begins and reduces the risk of hypoglycemia. Adjustment of the next meal bolus or the overnight basal rate may also be required as a consequence of increased muscle insulin sensitivity and the process of muscle glycogen repletion. Self-monitoring of blood glucose is essential in establishing specific responses and correctly anticipating therapeutic changes.

If the pump is put in Suspend mode while exercising, the pump user should be aware of the possibility that a clog may develop in the infusion set. It is therefore recommended that the Suspend mode be used for no more than two hours.

A useful starting point is to decrease the basal rate to half the usual infusion rate for the duration of the activity.

CASE STUDY 1

Megan K. is a 24-year old woman who has always been physically active and enjoys long-distance running. She has just run the Boston Marathon wearing her pump. Her training for the race included several weeks of careful monitoring of blood glucose levels. After a good night's rest and when she is under reasonable glycemic control, her blood glucose upon arising is 72 to 144 mg/dL. Her basal rate is 0.9 unit per hour. On the day of the marathon, she recorded a fasting blood glucose of 128 mg/dL. She ate a small breakfast after taking a small prebreakfast insulin bolus. Before starting the run, she reduced her basal rate to a temporary rate of 0.4 unit per hour. During the run, she took extra fluids and calories in the form of Gatorade every 30 to 45 minutes to maintain her fluid balance and energy level and to improve endurance. Her blood glucose values during the run were 81, 108 and 72 mg/dL. At the end of the race her blood glucose was in target range and she had not experienced any hypoglycemia. After the race, she ate a light meal containing 30 grams of carbohydrate preceded by a bolus that was 50 percent of her usual dose in order to prevent postexercise hypoglycemia. She knew from experience that after a long-distance run her usual basal rate would result in nocturnal hypoglycemia, so she used a temporary basal of 0.7 unit per hour (a 20 percent reduction of her normal rate) from 11 PM to 5 AM, after which she resumed her usual basal rate.

Bolus Insulin Modification

If exercise is being performed in the postprandial period (i.e., within one to three hours after a meal), reduction in the premeal boluses will likely be required. For example, an individual who takes a 12-unit bolus before dinner would reduce his premeal bolus by 50 percent, to 6 units, if he plans to play 50 minutes of tennis after dinner (9,10). Changes in the insulin regimen may not be required with strenuous short-term exercise. Hypoglycemia commonly occurs later in the day following exercise (up to 24 hours later), and subsequent basal or bolus dose modification may be required (11).

PUMP-OFF STRATEGIES

Excessive movement, activity or contact may require removing the insulin pump for certain activities. As a general principle, if the pump is to be removed for less than one hour, no insulin replacement is necessary. If the time off the pump will be from one to four hours, the pump user should give an insulin bolus via the pump before it is disconnected,* or by injection after the pump is removed. In the context of exercise, the bolus replacement dose will have to be modified to prevent hypoglycemia. A good starting point is to reduce by 50 percent the amount of insulin that would have been infused during the time off the pump.

CASE STUDY 2

Brandon F. is a 35-year old man who enjoys playing tennis after supper several times during the week. His tennis matches include a warm-up period of about an hour followed by an hour of actual playing. His usual premeal bolus for supper is 12 units, but on the days he plays tennis (which usually starts about an hour after he eats) he reduces his premeal bolus to 8 units. He established this algorithm by monitoring his responses to different bolus adjustments. He checks his blood glucose before and after playing, and at the end of the match eats a snack of 20 grams carbohydrate after a 2-unit bolus. He reduces his basal rate from 1.0 unit to 0.7 unit per hour from bedtime to morning (11 PM to 7 AM) in order to avoid nocturnal hypoglycemia. This regimen has worked quite well for him. If he decides to play tennis at a different time of day (e.g., on the weekends), he reduces the appropriate premeal bolus before the match.

---

* See Chapter 9, Everyday Management, for more information on disconnecting with the Quick Release™

USING AN INSULIN PUMP IN SPORTS ACTIVITIES

Physically active pump users report an increased satisfaction in their ability to pursue their favorite sports, knowing their blood glucose levels are under control. To facilitate pump use with exercise, the Quick Release™ can be used to temporarily disconnect from the pump. The SportGuard™ case (MiniMed®) can also be used, and allows pump users to fully enjoy their favorite sports without fear of damaging the pump.

With any sports activity, pump users should check blood glucose after periods of extended pump removal, and change the infusion set whenever an unexplained high blood glucose occurs. This is especially important when activities that occurred during pump removal may have caused the infusion set to become dislodged.

Water Sports

Although many pump users are initially concerned about taking part in water sports, these activities can be easily managed. The infusion set can be disconnected for up to one hour during water activities. For longer activities, the pump user can wear the SportGuard case on a belt. To prevent extra tension on the tubing, an extra piece of tape can be used to secure it.

During more vigorous water sports, such as surfing, diving, or water polo, the pump user may feel more comfortable removing the pump. This can be done either by using the Quick Release™ or completely disconnecting, as at the time of an infusion set change.

Contact Sports

Most sports can be safely enjoyed while wearing the insulin pump. However, contact sports such as basketball, football, hockey, etc., may require extra protection of the pump itself to prevent damage. Many pump users who participate in team sports have found that using wide or elastic tape to hold the pump in the small of the back or under protective padding helps prevent damage to the pump and injury to the pump wearer in case of collision. The SportGuard case offers an additional level of protection. In any type of vigorous physical activity, perspiration may cause the tape to become loose. If this occurs, the pump user should apply antiperspirant around (but not on) the insertion site and under the area that will be covered by tape or dressing

Skiing, Skating and Winter Sports

Insulin is sensitive to cold (freezing) temperatures and therefore care must be taken to protect the pump and tubing during winter sports. Winter sports clothing often involves layers; the insulin pump should be worn under an inner layer (in underwear or leotards) for best protection during extended exposure to extremely cold temperatures. Although this is inconvenient for delivering a pre-meal bolus, it helps to protect the pump from falls and cold temperatures.

Because winter sports utilize glucose more rapidly (activity plus extra calories to maintain body temperature), adjustments in basal and bolus doses may be needed. Frequent blood glucose testing is, therefore, important.

SUMMARY

Exercise has significant health-promoting effects, primarily related to the cardiovascular system and circulating lipoproteins. People with IDDM need to compensate for the immediate and delayed effects of exercise on the blood glucose. CSII permits convenient adjustment of basal and bolus insulin dosage, as appropriate, to maintain blood glucose in the target range during and after exercise. Physically active pump users report increased satisfaction in their ability to pursue their favorite sports without having to compromise glycemic control or risk weight gain from increased carbohydrate intake.

REFERENCES

1. Zinman B. Diabetes and exercise: Clinical implications. In: Alberti KGMM, Krall KP, eds. *The Diabetes Annual*, No.5. Amsterdam: Elsevier Science Publishers, BV; 1990:173-185.

2. American Diabetes Association. Diabetes and exercise. Position statement. *Diabetes Care* 1990;13:804-805.

3. Horton ES. Exercise and diabetes mellitus. *Med Clin North Am* 1988; 72:1301-1321.

4. Wallberg-Henriksson H. Exercise and diabetes mellitus. In: Holloszy JO, ed. *Exercise and Sport Science Reviews*. Baltimore:Williams & Wilkins; 1992;20:339-368.

5. Sutton JR. Metabolic responses to exercise in normal and diabetic individuals. In: Strauss RH, ed. *Sports Medicine*. Philadelphia, PA: WB Saunders; 1992:221-237.

6. Zinman B, Vranic M, Albisser AM, Leibel BS, Marliss EB. The role of insulin in the metabolic response to exercise in diabetic man. *Diabetes* 1979; 28(Suppl 1):76-81.

7. Zinman B, Murray FT, Vranic M, Albisser AM, Leibel BS, McClean PA, Marliss EB. Glucoregulation during moderate exercise in insulin treated diabetics. *J Clin Endocrinol Metab* 1977;45:641-652.

8. Mitchell TH, Abraham G, Schiffrin A, Leiter LA, Marliss EB. Hyperglycemia after intense exercise in IDDM subjects during continuous subcutaneous insulin infusion. *Diabetes Care* 1988;11:311.

9. Sonnenberg GE, Kemmer FW, Berger M. Exercise in type I (insulin-dependent) diabetic patients treated with continuous subcutaneous insulin infusion. *Diabetologia* 1990;33:696-703.

10. Schiffrin A, Parikh S. Accommodating planned exercise in type I diabetic patients on intensive treatment. *Diabetes Care* 1985;8:337-343.

11. MacDonald MJ. Postexercise late-onset hypoglycemia in insulin-dependent diabetic patients. *Diabetes Care* 1978;10:58.

CHAPTER AUTHORS

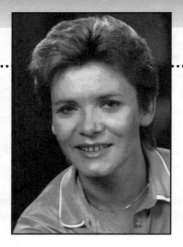

GABRIELE E. SONNENBERG, MD

Dr. Sonnenberg is Director of the Medical College of Wisconsin Diabetes Care Center, an American Diabetes Association-recognized center for diabetes patient education and treatment. She is also President of the Greater Milwaukee Chapter of the ADA. As one of the first physicians to begin using CSII therapy in Germany, Dr. Sonnenberg had built one of the largest insulin pump treatment centers in Europe before moving to the US. While intensive therapy and CSII continue to be the focus of her clinical work, her research activities, funded by both the NIH and industrial grants, focus on pancreatic beta-cell secretion in the normal and pathophysiologic state. She has authored more than 50 papers, reviews, and book chapters.

LINDA FREDRICKSON, MA, RN, CDE

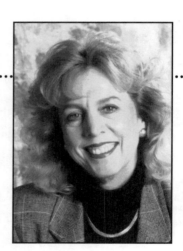

Linda Fredrickson is director of Professional Education and Clinical Services for MiniMed Technologies, Sylmar, CA. She has developed numerous pump therapy educational programs for patients and health care professionals in the US and abroad, including an innovative professional symposium series that has educated more than 2,500 physicians and nurses on insulin pump therapy and related technology. A long-time pump wearer, Ms. Fredrickson has been involved in the development and clinical testing of five generations of MiniMed insulin pumps. Before joining MiniMed, she served as an insulin pump project manager for Parker Biomedical, and as a diabetes research nurse at the University of Texas in Dallas. Ms. Fredrickson views her editorial role in *The Insulin Pump Therapy Book* as an excellent avenue for communicating to even more patients and health care professionals the knowledge and experience of some of the world's foremost authorities on insulin pump therapy.

DKA PREVENTION

11

Glucose derived from carbohydrate is the body's first choice as an energy source. Without insulin, cells cannot utilize glucose and the body shifts from metabolizing carbohydrate to fat for energy. This shift is accompanied by elevated blood glucose levels (hyperglycemia) and the appearance of normal, acidic by-products of fat metabolism known as ketones. When fats are the main source of energy, ketones accumulate and are detectable in the blood and urine. The accumulation of ketones moves the body's electrolyte balance to the acidic range, contributing to diuresis (excessive urination) and dehydration as the body tries to reestablish its acid-base balance by excreting the ketones. This life-threatening condition is known as diabetic ketoacidosis (DKA).

In people with type I diabetes, diabetic ketoacidosis can occur when the body's insulin requirement rises due to increased counterregulatory hormone action. This can occur, for example, with fever, infection, or unusual stress. In these situations, the increased insulin need must be matched with a greater insulin supply, whether the person is using injection therapy or continuous subcutaneous insulin infusion (CSII).

With CSII, technical problems that interfere with insulin delivery or absorption can cause DKA to develop rapidly even when insulin needs are no greater than usual. This can happen because there is no long-acting insulin present to act as a cushion or depot in the event of decreased insulin delivery (1). Complete interruption of insulin delivery may result in DKA within a period of four to eight hours (1,2); with partial interruption, DKA develops more slowly.

IN THIS CHAPTER

DKA Rates

Preventing DKA with Continuing Education

Prompt Response to Hyperglycemia

Potential Causes of Unexplained Hyperglycemia

The most common triggering event for DKA in all treatment protocols is failure to respond to elevated glucose readings immediately and appropriately.

Whether the result of increased insulin need, interrupted insulin delivery, or absorption difficulty, DKA can be prevented with appropriate action. Mecklenburg and colleagues observed that the most common triggering event for DKA in all treatment protocols is failure to respond to elevated blood glucose readings immediately and appropriately (1).

DKA RATES WITH CSII

Bending et al in the early years of pump use, reported comparable DKA rates between 40 pump users and 40 matched controls on conventional injection therapy (2). All episodes of DKA in the pump group occurred during the initial seven months of therapy. In five of the seven pump users who experienced DKA, failure to follow protocol (glucose monitoring, seeking help early and following advice, refilling the syringe) was a factor in the development of DKA.

Mecklenburg and associates reported an increase in the incidence of DKA in individuals who changed from conventional insulin therapy to CSII, and observed a higher rate of DKA in study participants on CSII (25 patients out of 161) versus those who remained on conventional therapy (6 patients out of 165) (1). In this study, individuals with DKA tended to have a higher mean glycosylated hemoglobin level and were younger than those without DKA. The majority (62%) of people who developed DKA while on pump therapy had their first episode within the first five months of pump therapy. Furthermore, in 50 percent of the DKA episodes, individuals had not checked for urine ketones or advanced their pump settings as instructed. More complete patient education in the beginning and increased experience with pump use played a role in reducing the risk of DKA in this study. Studies by Ronn (3), Chantelau (4), Wredling (5), and Bode (6) reported DKA rates of 6, 14, 10, and 7 episodes per 100 patient years, respectively. In all four studies, participants were given intensive training in diabetes self-management, including frequent blood glucose monitoring and DKA prevention, at the time of pump initiation.

Within the intensive treatment group of the Diabetes Control and Complications Trial (DCCT), DKA events were analyzed by predominant mode of therapy (CSII versus multiple daily injection). The incidence of DKA was more frequent in the CSII group than in the MDI group (1.8 vs. 0.8 events per 100 patient years). The higher rate of DKA in pump users may have been due to the learning curve involved as individuals and treatment centers began to use this new mode of therapy. As the study progressed, more patient education protocols were developed to promote prevention of DKA.

PREVENTING DKA DURING PUMP USE

Ongoing education, frequent self-monitoring of blood glucose (SMBG), and prompt action in the event of unexplained hyperglycemia are the keys to preventing the development of DKA in insulin pump users. A key concept is that diabetes must always be treated first, and causes of high blood glucose values investigated second. By following this rule, the pump user can prevent loss of control, accelerated DKA, unwanted hospitalizations, and morbidity/mortality.

Education

Prior to starting pump therapy, individuals must be educated to act quickly if they experience hyperglycemia. Intercurrent illness, infusion system leakage, and inflammation or infection at the infusion site are the most frequently reported precipitating causes of DKA in individuals using pumps. Less frequent causes, which should also be ruled out, include dislodgement of the cannula or needle, loss of insulin potency, poor absorption from the site, or an empty insulin reservoir. The importance of thorough training in sick-day management, skin care practices, and infusion set/pump techniques are underscored by these potential risks. Therefore, protocols should be developed by the health care team and pump user for preventing DKA during illness, insulin interruption, and other potentially problematic situations.

Despite thorough training and education, some pump users still experience DKA. Health care providers may become perplexed as to why DKA happens despite their having covered the subject so well during initiation. There are many reasons why pump users do not recognize the potential risk and therefore do not follow instructions when elevated blood glucose levels occur. In fact, it sometimes takes an episode of near-DKA for the pump user to become fully cognizant of the potential risk, and thus develop a healthy fear of DKA and a keen awareness of its early signs.

DKA prevention is usually taught at the time of pump initiation, when the pump user may already feel overloaded with information. Continuing DKA prevention education is, therefore, a must. Examples of DKA refresher questions for pump users are shown on the next page.

Regular Self-Monitoring Can Reveal Unexpected Hyperglycemia

Identification of elevated blood glucose levels can only be made through frequent blood glucose self-monitoring. Blood glucose levels should be monitored at least four times a day: upon awakening, and before lunch, dinner and bedtime. Periodically, blood glucose levels should also be checked at 3 AM. More frequent checks are required when illness or nausea is present.

Common Reasons Pump Users Fail To Treat Impending DKA

"It can't happen to me, I've had diabetes for 20 years."

"Everything had been perfect for four years of pump therapy."

"I was under a lot of stress."

"My girlfriend had the flu, I thought I caught it from her."

"These high blood sugars are my fault: I ate too much."

"I moved and forgot where the instructions were."

"I didn't have any Ketostix".

"I didn't have any regular insulin."

"DKA only happens to non-compliant patients."

Refresher Questions on DKA Prevention

1. Diabetic ketoacidosis (DKA) can occur more quickly in pump users.
   True ☐ False ☐

2. Pump users can help prevent DKA by taking an injection of regular insulin when blood glucose levels don't respond to a bolus.
   True ☐ False ☐

3. Whenever nausea and vomiting occur, the first likely cause is food poisoning.
   True ☐ False ☐

4. Most pump users who experience DKA feel they could have prevented the occurrence.
   True ☐ False ☐

5. DKA can be life-threatening.
   True ☐ False ☐

Unexplained hyperglycemia is defined as a high blood glucose level, usually discovered through routine monitoring, in the absence of known cause such as illness, changes in dietary intake, decreased insulin dosage, decreased level of activity or increased stress (8). If the blood glucose level increases even after administering a supplemental insulin dose, with or without the presence of urine ketones, it is likely that insulin delivery has been interrupted.

PROMPT ACTION IN THE EVENT OF HYPERGLYCEMIA

A quick response to hyperglycemia can prevent DKA. Whenever an insulin delivery problem is suspected, the pump user should change the reservoir, insulin, infusion set and site. If a cause of hyperglycemia is not found, it should be assumed that blockage has occurred, and the infusion set should be changed. Long-term pump users have learned to develop a low threshold for changing their tubing whenever unexplained hyperglycemia occurs (9).

Pump users with nausea, vomiting, or other symptoms of DKA (stomach upset, headache, muscle and joint aches) or blood glucose levels higher than 240 mg/dL should always check for the presence of urinary ketones. If urinary ketones are present or if the blood glucose level does not return to the target range within two to three hours after an infusion set change, the health care provider should be contacted immediately and a supplemental dose of regular insulin should be taken by subcutaneous injection using a syringe. If ketones are moderate to large, the supplemental dose may need to be increased by as much as 50 to 100 percent. This dose should be coordinated with the health care provider. In addition, the pump user may require injections of regular insulin every 60 to 120 minutes. It is very important in impending DKA to replace fluids with copious amounts of non-caloric fluids (16 ounces of water, tea, or broth every hour). The importance of fluid replacement should be stressed, because when ketones are present it may be hard for the pump user to consume these extra fluids due to nausea.

When the blood glucose level falls below 200 mg/dL, the insulin dosage should be reduced and fluid replacement with glucose-containing fluids (cola or a sports drink such as Gatorade) should continue.

If vomiting occurs, the pump user should notify the health care provider immediately and begin giving all insulin by syringe. If blood glucose is still high and no oral fluid intake is possible, the pump user must be seen in the Emergency Room for intravenous fluid replacement. It has been shown, however, that if the pump user contacts the health care provider early, he or she is usually able to manage the hyperglycemia at home, saving an emergency room visit or hospitalization (9)

Supplies for insulin injection must always be kept on hand, and pump users must know when to inject and how much insulin to administer by injection.

Additional pump supplies (batteries, infusion sets, and pump syringes) are essential for the pump user, in case a problem with insulin delivery develops. In an emergency, the insulin in the pump reservoir (after the catheter is disconnected from the body and the pump) can be used for an injection by withdrawing it with a conventional syringe.

POSSIBLE CAUSES OF HYPERGLYCEMIA

Infusion set occlusion or leak

Pump users are encouraged to adhere to a regular schedule for changing the infusion set and filling the insulin reservoir. Routine infusion set changes should be made every 48 to 72 hours, preferably in the morning, and immediately before administering a bolus dose. When connecting a new infusion set, the pump user must ensure that the tubing is properly primed. If blood appears in the tubing, the infusion set should be replaced right away to prevent blockage of insulin delivery due to blood clot formation. The blood glucose level should always be measured three hours after inserting a new infusion set to ensure proper insulin delivery.

The pump user must check for leaks when changing the reservoir and infusion set, whenever he or she smells insulin, or whenever unexplained high blood glucose levels are present. As a routine check for leaks, the pump user, while manually filling the infusion set, should place his or her fingers on the luer junction between the syringe and infusion set to make certain there are no leaks. Leaks in the infusion tubing cannot be detected by the pump alarm system, and are most often discovered by way of an unexplained high blood glucose level.

Insulin occlusions in the infusion tubing may appear as white crystalline deposits or merely as insulin adhering to the side of the tubing. A partial clog does not activate the pump alarm until sufficient pressure has built up and the line is totally occluded, which can take several hours. An unexplained high blood glucose level is often the first sign of an occlusion. To check for clogs, the pump user should remove the infusion set and give a bolus into the air. If the insulin does not immediately appear at the tip, the infusion set is clogged and should be replaced with a new infusion set. Reinsertion of the used infusion set should not be allowed because of the increased risk of staphylococcal contamination (10).

To minimize clogging, insulin-compatible (polyolefin) infusion tubing is recommended. The infusion set should be inserted prior to administration of a bolus to lessen the possibility that tissue will clog the cannula or needle (8).

Reservoir

The pump user is advised to check the amount of insulin remaining in the reservoir at least once a day. An empty reservoir will be signaled by a "No Delivery"

The pump user must check for leaks when changing the reservoir and infusion set, and whenever unexplained high blood glucose levels are present.

Pump User's Guide to DKA Prevention

1. Monitor blood glucose levels at least 4 times a day, including bedtime. An unexplained high blood glucose level is often the first sign of interrupted insulin delivery.

2. Monitor blood glucose and urine ketones more frequently on sick days.

3. Check the infusion site, set, and reservoir. Follow precautions to prevent leakage or obstruction in the infusion set. Refill reservoir as needed and change infusion set if there is any question about proper insulin delivery, especially at bedtime!

4. Treat hyperglycemia promptly to prevent DKA. Test for urinary ketones at the first sign of nausea or if the blood glucose level is greater than 240 mg/dL.

alarm and should be refilled immediately. The insulin remaining in the tubing will not be infused into the body, as the syringe plunger has been pushed to its maximum. Therefore, pump users should not run down to the "last drop" because, even though the pump alarm will sound, delivery could be deficient by one or two units. On general principle it is best to plan ahead and change the reservoir before it runs out of insulin.

Insulin

Insulin that is cloudy, beyond its expiration date, or that has been exposed to temperature extremes should not be used. The potential for decreased insulin strength exists if insulin is exposed to low or high temperatures, either while still in the vial or after transfer to the pump reservoir. This can happen, for example, if the pump user goes sunbathing and forgets to shade the pump, or if he or she leaves insulin in a briefcase in a car or packs it in checked baggage on an airplane. Ordering insulin via mail order supply houses raises the risk that it will be exposed to temperature extremes during shipping, or while it sits in the pump user's mailbox.

Infusion Sets

When pump use first became popular in the early 1980s, infusion sets made of a polyvinylchloride (PVC) type of material were the primary cause of infusion set clogging (11). PVC allows gases, such as carbon dioxide (CO_2), to pass through relatively easily. When CO_2 gas dissolves in insulin, it can lower the pH and contribute to insulin precipitation and the possibility of clogging. Dissolved CO_2 can also cause a decrease in insulin strength. PVC infusion sets are known to leach additives into solution that can react with insulin and chemically bind the insulin molecules to the surface of the tubing. This binding can result in a decrease in insulin strength.

Infusion sets (such as MiniMed Technologies' Polyfin™ and Sof-set™) lined with a insulin-compatible material such as polyolefin plastic have been shown to reduce the incidence of clogs (12). Before the advent of these insulin-compatible tubings, the medical community felt the only way to prevent "clogging" was to use buffered insulin (13). While many physicians recommend the use of buffered insulin in the pump, others successfully use unbuffered insulins. Any change in the type of insulin used in a pump should be made cautiously and should include extra blood glucose testing.

Infusion Sites

A hematoma at the infusion site, signaled by a lump under the skin, discomfort at the infusion site, or blood in the infusion line, will interfere with insulin delivery and absorption. If subcutaneous bleeding is suspected, the pump user should replace the infusion set and relocate the site to give the site with the hematoma time to heal.

Perspiration increases the chance of the tape becoming loose, which can lead to dislodgement of the cannula or needle. Therefore, pump users should check the infusion set and tape after exercise or other periods of increased activity or perspiration.

Incorrect Programming

The pump user should verify that the basal rate(s) is properly programmed and that any temporary basal rates have not been set and forgotten (despite the hourly reminder beeps). In addition, he or she should review the last several meal boluses to ensure that they were given correctly. High blood glucose levels can be caused by failure to program an adequate meal bolus or eating too soon after taking a meal bolus, especially if the blood glucose was elevated before the meal (see Chapter 6, *Bolus & Supplemental Insulin*). Pump users must take appropriate insulin boluses to match to the carbohydrate content of each meal.

Interruption in Pump Delivery

Pumps today have very sophisticated safety systems which will sound an alarm to signal malfunction, low battery, or stoppage or interruption of insulin delivery. One of the most important technological safety advances in insulin pumps is the presence of a high pressure or occlusion alarm. This alarm (also called a "No Delivery Alarm") will sound when the pump detects that the plunger arm cannot move forward for any reason. Health care providers and pump users should learn to test the pump's occlusion alarm by clamping off the tubing after the pump has been primed and giving a bolus. Not all pumps have an occlusion alarm of the same sensitivity. One pump (MiniMed 506) will alarm within two to four units of missed insulin when the infusion set is completely blocked, while a pump with a less sensitive alarm may not alarm until nine to ten units have been missed. In clinical practice, if a pump user with a basal rate of 1.0 unit per hour goes to bed at 10 PM, a sensitive alarm will occur between midnight and 2 AM if the infusion set becomes clogged, while a less sensitive alarm may not occur until morning. If the pump is delivering a low basal rate, for example, 0.3 unit per hour, the delay becomes even more critical.

Pump users should not wait for the pump to alert them to a problem, as even the most sensitive occlusion alarms will not activate unless the tubing is completely blocked. If inaccurate insulin delivery is suspected, the pump user should verify delivery using the lead screw test described in the *User's Guide*. If a pump malfunction is confirmed, the pump user should contact his or her health care provider and/or the pump manufacturer immediately.

Pump User's Guide to DKA Prevention
continued

5. Take a supplemental dose of regular insulin by injection whenever urinary ketones are present or blood glucose levels do not respond to an infusion set change within 2 to 3 hours. Contact your health care provider.

6. If urinary ketones are moderate or large increase the supplemental insulin dose by 50 to 100 percent. Drink at least 8 ounces of water or other non-caloric beverage every 30 minutes and test blood glucose levels at least every hour until blood glucose returns to the target range.

7. Supplemental insulin doses should be given by syringe until the cause of nausea or hyperglycemia is identified and treated.

POTENTIAL CAUSES OF UNEXPLAINED HYPERGLYCEMIA
adapted from Strowig (8)

1. Insulin pump
- Basal rate programmed incorrectly
- Pump malfunction; improperly advancing reservoir
- Program/pump alarms
- Insensitive occlusion alarm

2. Reservoir
- Improper placement in pump
- Empty syringe
- Insulin leakage at luer lock

3. Infusion set/needle
- Infusion set not primed
- Insulin leakage
- Needle or cannula dislodged
- Air in infusion set (tiny bubbles will not affect blood glucose control, 1 inch of air = 1/2 unit of insulin)
- Blood in infusion set
- Infusion set in over 48 hours
- Infusion set inserted at bedtime and no bolus given
- Kinked tubing
- Catheter occlusion

4. Infusion site
- Redness, irritation, inflammation
- Discomfort
- Area of hypertrophy or scar tissue
- Area of friction on or near the belt line, leading to infusion set dislodgement

5. Insulin
- Cloudy
- Beyond expiration date
- Exposed to temperature extremes

SUMMARY

To avoid DKA, a pump user must be thoroughly educated in the importance of frequent blood glucose monitoring, troubleshooting high blood glucose levels, and the protocol for pump discontinuation in the event of impending DKA. Daily checks of the entire infusion system (reservoir volume and placement, tubing and infusion site integrity, basal and bolus programming, etc.) can be helpful in identifying and avoiding potential episodes of DKA.

Prompt action in the case of a suspected interruption in insulin delivery can help prevent the development of DKA. By the time insulin interruption is discovered, it usually has been occurring for several hours. Simply restarting the insulin infusion may not be enough to prevent DKA. Extra insulin should be given until blood glucose is returned to normal. The extra insulin should be given by means of syringe whenever a pump user experiences vomiting, when ketones are present, or when elevated blood glucose levels do not respond to boluses via the pump.

Knowledgeable and motivated pump users can expect to experience no greater incidence of DKA than those using insulin injection therapy.

Knowledgeable and motivated pump users can expect to experience no greater incidence of DKA than those using insulin injection therapy.

REFERENCES

1. Mecklenburg RS, Benson EA, Benson JW, Fredlund PN, Guinn T, Metz RJ, Nielsen RL, Sannar CA. Acute complications associated with insulin infusion pump therapy. Report of experience with 161 patients. JAMA 1984;252:3265-3269.

2. Bending J, Pickup JC, Keen H. The frequency of diabetic ketoacidosis and hypoglycemic coma during treatment with continuous subcutaneous insulin infusion. *Am J Med* 1985;79:685-691.

3. Ronn B, Mathiesen ER, Vang L, Lorup B, Deckert T. Evaluation of insulin pump treatment under routine conditions. *Diabetes Res Clin Pract* 1989;3:191-196.

4. Chantelau E, Spraul M, Muhlhauser I, Gause R, Berger M. Long-term safety, efficacy and side effects of continuous subcutaneous insulin infusion treatment for type I (insulin dependent) diabetes mellitus: a one centre experience. *Diabetologia* 1989;32:421-426.

5. Wredling R, Lins PE, Adamson U. Factors influencing the clinical outcome of continuous subcutaneous insulin infusion in routine practice. *Diabetes Res Clin Pract* 1993;19:59-67.

6. Bode B, Steed D, Davidson P. Long-term pump use and SMBG in 205 patients. *Diabetes* 1994;43(Suppl 1):220A.

7. The Diabetes Control and Complications Trial Research Group. The effect of intensive treatment of diabetes on the development and progression of long-term complications in insulin-dependent diabetes mellitus. *N Engl J Med* 1993;329:977-986.

8. Strowig SM. Initiation and management of insulin pump therapy. *Diabetes Educ* 1993;19:50-59.

9. Farkas-Hirsch R, Hirsch IB. Continuous subcutaneous insulin infusion: a review of the past and its implementation for the future. *Diabetes Spectrum* 1994;7:80-84.

10. Chantelau E, Lange G, Sonnenberg GE, Berger M. Acute cutaneous complications and catheter needle colonization during insulin-pump treatment. *Diabetes Care* 1987;10:478-482.

11. Hirsch JI, Wood JH, Thomas RB. Insulin adsorption to polyolefin infusion bottles and polyvinylchloride administration sets. *Am J Hosp Pharm* 1981;38:995-997.

12. Drazin RL, Van Antwerp W, Konopka A, Lord P, Fredrickson L. Comparison of PVC and polyolefin catheters for insulin compatibility during continuous subcutaneous insulin infusion (CSII). *Diabetes* 1986;35:140A.

13. Mecklenburg R, Guinn T. Complications of insulin pump therapy: the effect of insulin preparation. *Diabetes Care* 1985;8:367-370.

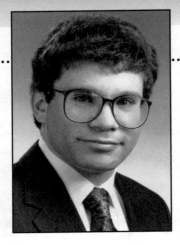

Irl B. Hirsch, MD

Irl B. Hirsch is Associate Professor of Medicine and Medical Director of the Diabetes Care Center at the University of Washington, Seattle, WA. His research is focused on various aspects of intensive therapy, including hypoglycemia and implementation of CSII. Other interests include perioperative and inpatient diabetes management, strategies for the screening and treatment of diabetic nephropathy, and most recently, oxidative modifications of LDL cholesterol in diabetes. Dr. Hirsch is active in the American Diabetes Association both locally and nationally, and lectures throughout the US. He has worn an insulin pump for more than a decade.

William H. Polonsky, PhD, CDE

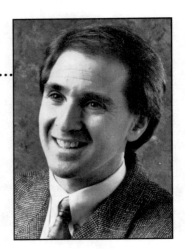

William H. Polonsky is a licensed clinical psychologist and a certified diabetes educator. Currently, he is staff psychologist at Sharp HealthCare Diabetes Management and Treatment Center in San Diego, and also maintains a private practice, specializing in psychosocial issues of diabetes. Dr. Polonsky has served as chairman of the National Certification Board for Diabetes Educators, Senior Psychologist at the Joslin Diabetes Center in Boston, and Instructor in Psychiatry at Harvard Medical School. An active researcher, he has authored a wide range of professional articles on psychosocial and behavioral issues in diabetes.

HYPOGLYCEMIA AND ITS PREVENTION

12

Hypoglycemia is always a risk for those receiving insulin. The risk of hypoglycemia associated with intensive therapy is a reflection of the degree of glycemic control (1) and whether the person's counterregulatory responses are intact (2). Continuous subcutaneous insulin infusion (CSII), with its more predictable delivery of insulin, may reduce the incidence of severe hypoglycemia, even in individuals with a history of severe hypoglycemia or reduced hypoglycemic awareness (3-9).

SIGNS AND SYMPTOMS OF HYPOGLYCEMIA

Neurogenic (sometimes referred to as autonomic) symptoms of impending hypoglycemia are mediated by adrenergic and cholinergic mechanisms. These symptoms are summarized in Table 1. Based on these symptoms, hypoglycemic episodes are generally categorized as presymptomatic (biochemical), mild-moderate, or severe (11).

Presymptomatic or biochemical hypoglycemia is detected only by measurement of the blood glucose concentration. Typically, the blood glucose level falls through this presymptomatic phase to the mild-moderate phase before symptoms of hypoglycemia become apparent. Mild-moderate hypoglycemic reactions are characterized by symptoms such as tremors, tingling, palpitations, diaphoresis (sweating) and excessive hunger. Cognitive functions may also be impaired, although such changes often go unnoticed by the individual or a casual observer. In mild-moderate hypoglycemia, the person experiencing the hypoglycemic episode can usually recognize and treat the symptoms without outside help.

IN THIS CHAPTER

Dangers of Hypoglycemia

Rates of Hypoglycemia with CSII

Reduced Hypoglycemic Awareness

Blood Glucose Awareness Training

Any form of hypoglycemia is potentially dangerous. It has been reported that 4% of all deaths in people with diabetes result from hypoglycemia.

> **Table 1**
>
> ## COMMON SYMPTOMS OF HYPOGLYCEMIA
>
> | *Neurogenic* | *Neuroglycopenic* | *Miscellaneous* |
> |---|---|---|
> | Sweating | Dizziness | Hunger |
> | Tremors | Confusion | Blurred vision |
> | Anxiety | Headache | |
> | Nausea | Speech impairment | |
> | Palpitations | Drowsiness | |
> | Shivering | Weakness | |
>
> Adapted from Towler, et al (10)

Severe hypoglycemia is associated with marked neuroglycopenia (impaired cognitive function that results directly from brain glucose deprivation) and may lead to unresponsiveness, coma, or seizure. As defined by the Diabetes Control and Complications Trial (DCCT), severe hypoglycemia requires assistance from another person for appropriate treatment (1).

DANGERS OF HYPOGLYCEMIA

Any form of hypoglycemia is potentially dangerous. It has been reported that four percent of all deaths in people with diabetes result from hypoglycemia (12). Situations requiring quick reaction or judgement, such as the safe operation of a motor vehicle, can be compromised even in mild hypoglycemic episodes. Two fatal motor vehicle accidents in which hypoglycemia may have had a causative role were reported in the DCCT. In addition, a third person who was not involved in the DCCT was killed by a driver who was a participant in the trial and thought to be hypoglycemic (1). Cox and colleagues have also reported that moderate hypoglycemia interfered with the operation of a motor vehicle and was associated with more erratic steering, swerving, spinning, time over the midline, and time off the road (13). Moderate hypoglycemia can also result in very slow driving, which can be quite dangerous on a busy freeway.

Several studies have addressed the issue of whether long-term neurologic damage can be caused by repeated episodes of severe hypoglycemia. Deary et al revealed a small, cumulative detrimental effect on performance IQ in patients with a history of severe hypoglycemia (14). Wredling and associates observed some cognitive impairment that was thought to result from repeated episodes of hypoglycemia (15). Reichard and colleagues reported no hypoglycemia-related cognitive damage over a five-year period, although they used neuropsychological tests that are unlikely to be sensitive to mild cognitive impairment (16,17). Impaired visual/spatial cognitive functions directly related to the frequency of mild hypoglycemia have been reported in children diagnosed with IDDM before the age of four or five years (18).

Nocturnal Hypoglycemia

Over 50 percent of all episodes of severe hypoglycemia occur during sleep (19). Nocturnal hypoglycemia is often asymptomatic. Indeed, unrecognized nocturnal hypoglycemia may be relatively common, occurring in at least one-third (or greater) of those with IDDM. If symptoms do occur, they may not arouse someone from sleep, which can allow a mild hypoglycemic episode to progress to a more severe situation because of lack of treatment (20). A contributing factor to the relatively high frequency of severe hypoglycemia during the night may be that persons with IDDM tend to be less aware of symptoms of hypoglycemia when lying down as compared to when standing (21). Perhaps even more important is the fact that insulin sensitivity is greatest, and thus insulin requirements are least, in the middle of the night (22).

Fear of nocturnal hypoglycemia can lead to chronic hyperglycemia if the pump user overcompensates for moderate to low blood glucose values at bedtime by increasing carbohydrate intake or reducing insulin doses (23). Such a pattern may, in turn, affect glycemic control throughout the day (24). Use of an insulin pump allows programmed reductions in basal insulin delivery during periods of decreased insulin need, such as the nighttime hours, and helps to prevent nocturnal hypoglycemia (22).

Rates of Severe Hypoglycemia with Insulin Pump Therapy

The DCCT revealed that severe hypoglycemia can be a significant problem in individuals using intensive therapy to maintain near-normal blood glucose levels. In the DCCT, severe hypoglycemia occurred at the rate of 62 events per 100 patient years in those using intensive therapy administered by pump or multiple daily injections (MDI). This rate was threefold higher than that experienced by participants in the conventionally-treated group. Fifty-five percent of severe hypoglycemic events occured during sleep, with 43 percent of severe events occurring between midnight and 8 AM. Over one-third (36 percent) of the severe hypoglycemic episodes in the DCCT occurred while subjects were awake and were not accompanied by warning symptoms (25).

A subsequent analysis of the DCCT data compared the participants who used either MDI or CSII at least 90 percent of the time (26). This analysis revealed that CSII users achieved a lower mean HbA_{1c} (6.8 percent vs 7.0 percent, p < 0.05), but had no greater incidence of severe hypoglycemia than those using

Use of an insulin pump allows programmed reductions in basal insulin delivery during periods of decreased insulin need, such as the nighttime hours, and helps to prevent nocturnal hypoglycemia.

MDI. However, the frequency of severe hypoglycemic episodes that resulted in coma or seizure was higher in the CSII group (18 events per 100 patient years) than in the MDI group (10 episodes per 100 patient years).

Table 2

COMPARISON OF SEVERE HYPOGLYCEMIA AND GLYCEMIC CONTROL DURING LONG-TERM (>1 YEAR) CSII USE

Investigator (reference)	Number of Patients	Mean Observation Time (Years)	Total Patient Years	Severe Hypoglycemia (per 100 patient years)	HbA$_{1c}$ (percent)	HbA$_{1c}$ Normal Range (percent)
Bode (3)	205	2.9	>600	28	7.2	3.4-6.1
Mecklenburg (27)	161	1.5	248	*7	8.8	4.5-8.0
DCCT (26)	124	≥4.5	761	54	6.8	4.5-6.0
Chantelau (5)	116	4.5	518	10	6.7	4.8±0.3
Ronn (4)	66	1.6	130	9	7.5	4.1-6.4
Wredling (6)	49	3.5	130	25	7.6	4.0-5.6
Bell** (8)	55	8.4		20	8.3	5.5-8.5
Eichner** (7)	45	2.4		22	8.1	4.0-7.9

* Hypoglycemic coma only

**Retrospective study

Other long-term studies of CSII have demonstrated excellent glycemic control with lower rates of severe hypoglycemia than the DCCT (Table 2). Mecklenburg et al found no significant change in the rate of hypoglycemic coma from the pre-CSII year, when study participants used conventional insulin treatment, to the CSII treatment period (27). In a retrospective study, Eichner et al reported a marked decrease in severe hypoglycemia when participants changed from MDI (273 events per 100 patient years) to CSII (22 events per 100 patient years) (7). Bode and colleagues also observed a significant reduction in the rate of severe hypoglycemia during pump therapy (28 events per 100 patient years) as compared to the prepump year when injection-based insulin therapy was used (182 events per 100 patient years) (3). The reasons for the difference in results between these studies and the DCCT are not clear.

Causes and Prevention of Hypoglycemia on CSII

As seen in the DCCT, people using insulin who strive for normal to near-normal blood glucose levels may be subject to increased risk for hypoglycemia. Raising blood glucose target goals in individuals who have a history of severe hypoglycemia or reduced hypoglycemic awareness is an important principle of

Table 3
CAUSES AND PREVENTION OF HYPOGLYCEMIA WITH PUMP THERAPY

Cause	Prevention
Inappropriate target blood glucose levels.	Set target blood glucose ranges higher for pump users with a history of hypoglycemia or reduced hypoglycemia awareness.
Basal rate set too high.	Confirm appropriateness of basal rate(s). If hypoglycemia occurs when meals are delayed, an adjustment in basal rate is needed. Periodically measure blood glucose at 3 AM to determine whether overnight basal rate needs to be reduced.
Taking too large a bolus for the carbohydrate content of a meal.	Provide specific, individualized guidelines for meal-related boluses.
Not compensating for exercise by making appropriate adjustments in insulin dose and/or food intake. Unusually long or intense exercise can cause delayed (post-exercise) hypoglycemia.	Instruct pump users to compensate for exercise with appropriate decreases in basal or bolus insulin doses or increased carbohydrate intake. Administer bedtime boluses with extreme caution after unusually intense or prolonged exercise.
Excessive bolusing to correct hyperglycemia.	Provide specific, individualized guidelines for supplemental insulin doses (Refer to the "1500 Rule," Chapter 6). Before bolusing, pump user may use pump memory feature to review all boluses given in the previous 5 hours.
Insufficient frequency of blood glucose monitoring.	Instruct pump users to monitor at least 4 times a day, including bedtime. Less frequent monitoring does not allow prompt enough response to an out-of-range level.
Drinking alcohol.	Warn pump users about the hypoglycemic effect of alcohol. Individuals should administer bedtime boluses with extreme caution after drinking alcohol.

intensive diabetes management, whether with CSII or multiple daily injections. For example, a person with diabetes and no history of severe hypoglycemia may have a target premeal blood glucose of 70 to 150 mg/dL, while an individual with recurrent severe hypoglycemia could aim at a level in the range of 100 to 200 mg/dL.

Insulin pump users typically experience less extreme swings in blood glucose levels and fewer or more subtle symptoms of low blood glucose. This is because CSII eliminates the considerable variation in absorption and the unpredictable postprandial peaks that can occur with modified insulins (28). Pump users must guard against hypoglycemia by monitoring blood glucose levels at least four times a day, including bedtime, **and** whenever they suspect hypoglycemia. To prevent severe hypoglycemia, out-of-range blood glucose levels should always be treated promptly, whether or not symptoms are felt.

It has been shown that the frequency of nocturnal hypoglycemia can be significantly reduced if bedtime blood glucose values are greater than 100 mg/dL (29). At least once a week, the pump user should test in the middle of the night (i.e., between 1 AM and 4 AM) to ensure that overnight insulin delivery rates are appropriate and nocturnal hypoglycemia is not occurring.

TREATMENT OF HYPOGLYCEMIA

People with diabetes should keep fast-acting carbohydrate with them at all times and know how to calculate the proper dose for raising the blood glucose level sufficiently without overtreating. For most people, 5 grams of fast-acting carbohydrate will raise the blood glucose by about 20 mg/dL. For example, a person needing to raise his or her blood glucose by 60 mg/dL would take 15 grams of carbohydrate. This formula can be fine-tuned based on a person's body weight.

All individuals using insulin, including those using CSII, should have a Glucagon Emergency Kit. Family members should be trained in using it, and the telephone number of the health care provider should be kept in the kit. Family members may be reluctant to use glucagon if they are not familiar with its use, and will need reassurance from the diabetes team that no harm will be done in administering it to their loved one. It is the pump user's responsibility to inform family members where the glucagon is stored. This is especially true after a change in residence, or after a trip where the kit might have been placed in a travel bag. One should mark the kit's expiration date on the calendar as a reminder to replace it with a fresh one.

SEVERE, PERSISTENT HYPOGLYCEMIA

If severe or persistent hypoglycemia occurs, it may indicate that insulin dosing is incorrect or that the basic principles of blood glucose control are not understood or are not being followed. Evaluate the pump user's understanding and application of the following guidelines, and correct any deficiencies:

- The basal rate(s) and bolus dosages must be correct
  (See Chapters 5, *Establishing & Verifying Basal Rates*, and Chapter 6, *Bolus & Supplemental Insulin*).

Some people pursuing tight blood glucose control tend to minimize the seriousness of low blood glucose values, being much more concerned and/or even fearful about high values.

- Carbohydrate counting should be used to assure accurate boluses (See Chapter 7, *Counting Carbohydrates*).

- The correct supplemental dose, based on the person's sensitivity to insulin, must be used to correct high blood glucose levels (refer to the "1500 Rule" and "Calculating the Supplemental Dose" in Chapter 6, *Bolus & Supplemental Insulin*). People differ in their sensitivity to insulin, and a supplement that brings one person's blood glucose into the target range may send another's too low. Many insulin users have reported hypoglycemic events that were caused by overbolusing in response to a high blood glucose level. Determining the correct supplemental dose is as important as determining the correct basal rate and premeal bolus doses in preventing hypoglycemia.

It is also important to assess an individual's attitudes about the acceptability of high and low blood glucose values. Such an assessment might begin with the question, "What is more acceptable, a blood glucose of 50 mg/dL or a blood glucose of 220 mg/dL?" Some people pursuing tight blood glucose control tend to minimize the seriousness of low blood glucose values, being much more concerned and/or even fearful about high values. Those with such an unreasonable fear of hyperglycemia may be placing themselves at greater risk for hypoglycemia by not taking appropriate preventive measures.

REDUCED HYPOGLYCEMIC AWARENESS

Reduced hypoglycemic awareness is defined as an impairment in the ability to recognize symptoms of developing hypoglycemia, such as tremors, palpitations and sweating, that previously prompted intake of carbohydrate (30). This syndrome is often referred to as "hypoglycemic unawareness," however the loss of symptom awareness is rarely total. For example, mood changes and some neuroglycopenic symptoms are often still present, but go unnoticed. Reduced hypoglycemic awareness can allow significant mental impairment to occur before hypoglycemia is recognized (2). A clinical history of reduced hypoglycemic awareness is known to result in a five- to sixfold increase in the frequency of severe hypoglycemia in persons with IDDM (31,32).

CAUSES OF REDUCED HYPOGLYCEMIC AWARENESS OR SYMPTOMS

Compromised Glucose Counterregulation

Glucose counterregulation (glucose-raising) is a mechanism that helps prevent or correct hypoglycemia through the activation of glucose counterregulatory hormones such as glucagon and epinephrine. This system is normally activated at blood glucose levels higher than those at which most symptoms of hypoglycemia occur. Glucagon is the body's first defense against hypoglycemia; epinephrine is not necessary when glucagon is present but becomes critical to glucose counterregulation when glucagon is deficient (11).

Meticulous avoidance of all hypoglycemia resulted in increased symptomatic responses to hypoglycemia after two weeks, and normalization of the responses after three months.

A single episode of hypoglycemia (blood glucose less than 70 mg/dL) has been shown to reduce glucagon and epinephrine secretions and neurogenic responses to hypoglycemia over the next 24 to 72 hours.

Glucagon secretion typically becomes deficient in nearly everyone with IDDM within the first two to five years after diabetes onset (2). A reduced epinephrine response may develop later in the course of IDDM. Other counterregulatory hormones such as cortisol and growth hormone are not adequate, even under normal circumstances, to prevent hypoglycemia. Therefore, persons with combined deficiencies in their glucagon and epinephrine responses have little defense, other than scrupulous prevention, against severe hypoglycemia (9,31).

Recent studies have demonstrated that reduced hypoglycemic awareness may be reversible. Fanelli et al found that meticulous avoidance of all hypoglycemia resulted in increased symptomatic responses to hypoglycemia after two weeks, and normalization of the responses after three months, in IDDM patients with a history of reduced hypoglycemic awareness (33). Dagogo-Jack and colleagues demonstrated a similar reversal (30). A later study by the Fanelli group confirmed and strengthened their original findings and also indicated that long-term (at least one year) maintenance of recovery from reduced hypoglycemic awareness is possible (34).

Conflicting results have been reported, however, regarding the reversibility of defective counterregulation. In the Fanelli studies, increased, although not normalized, epinephrine and glucagon secretions were observed during the avoidance of hypoglycemia (33,34). Dagogo-Jack and associates saw no such increases, leading them to conclude that the mechanisms of reduced hypoglycemic awareness and defective glucose counterregulation are, at least partially, separate in IDDM (30).

Antecedent Hypoglycemia
When an insulin user has had a hypoglycemic episode, the risk of his having a subsequent episode is increased. A single episode of hypoglycemia (blood glucose less than 70 mg/dL) has been shown to reduce glucagon and epinephrine secretions and neurogenic responses to hypoglycemia over the next 24 to 72 hours, even in individuals with IDDM who have no history of severe hypoglycemia (35-37). The resulting cycle of recurrent hypoglycemia can be difficult to break and can result in defective counterregulation and reduced awareness of neurogenic symptoms. This combination has been described as hypoglycemia-associated autonomic failure, a clinical disorder unrelated to diabetic autonomic neuropathy (32,38). Glycemic thresholds for hypoglycemic symptoms may change after just one hypoglycemic episode in both nondiabetic individuals (39) and those with IDDM (40).

Drug-mediated Symptom Reduction
The perception of impending hypoglycemia is mediated, in part, by adrenergic mechanisms. These mechanisms and the resulting neurogenic symptoms of hypoglycemia may be blunted by drugs known as beta-adrenergic antagonists (beta-blockers), which are used in the treatment of certain cardiovascular disor-

ders, including hypertension. With use of beta-blockers, neurogenic symptoms diminish at blood glucose levels below 70 to 80 mg/dL, and diaphoresis can increase dramatically at the more dangerous blood glucose level of 50 mg/dL (41). To reduce the risk of severe hypoglycemia, an insulin user who takes beta-blockers should increase the frequency of routine blood glucose self-monitoring and perform extra self-testing whenever unexpected sweating occurs.

BLOOD GLUCOSE AWARENESS TRAINING

Now that the DCCT has demonstrated the value of normoglycemia as a target, programs will be needed to reduce the risk of hypoglycemia. Blood glucose awareness training (BGAT) is a relatively new, psychoeducational program to help people with diabetes avoid hypoglycemia without compromising glycemic control. This program uses a learning-by-doing approach to improve a person's ability to recognize subtle symptoms of hypoglycemia and to predict and treat low blood glucose levels (42,43). It also improves participants' understanding of the consequences of frequent hypoglycemia.

The seven-session BGAT program helps participants to increase their awareness of both internal (neurogenic, neuroglycopenic, mood shifts) and external (insulin, exercise, food) cues that may signal shifts in blood glucose levels. Regarding symptom perception in hypoglycemia, BGAT emphasizes two key facts:

1. Following a hypoglycemic episode, neurogenic symptoms may be significantly impaired for the next 24 hours, but neuroglycopenic symptoms remain mostly intact.

2. Even with adequate awareness, neurogenic symptoms may go unnoticed or be ignored due to extreme arousal or anxiety, distraction, and/or attributing them to other causes.

One session, for example, focuses on neuroglycopenic symptoms, referred to as "performance" cues. Initially, neuroglycopenic cues (e.g. concentration problems) may be very subtle. People can adapt easily and automatically to their occurrence, making awareness of their presence less likely. During this session, the wide range of possible neuroglycopenic symptoms is reviewed and participants are prompted to recall instances when there may have been subtle impairments, possibly blood glucose-related (e.g., slowed thinking, difficulty concentrating, or feeling uncoordinated), in their thoughts and/or actions. The goal is to sensitize these participants to the emergence of subtle neuroglycopenic symptoms, which can occur even during mild hypoglycemia, and to help them develop specific hypotheses about the association between blood glucose level and such symptoms. Participants test their hypotheses over the ensuing weeks through use of detailed blood glucose diaries.

BGAT Strategies For the Office or Clinic

- Negotiate a number, not a feeling, at which low blood glucose should be treated.

- Ask pump users to test their ability to estimate low blood glucose levels by recording estimated and actual blood glucose values for at least 2 weeks.

- Investigate pump users' beliefs concerning blood glucose-related symptoms, which are often innacurate (e.g., "whenever I feel hungry I know I'm low").

- Prompt pump users regarding all possible internal and external cues, giving special attention to neuroglycopenic cues, idiosyncratic cues and physical activity.

- Be aware that interpersonal relationships may be strained by hypoglycemic episodes, and offer counseling.

- Encourage participation in BGAT seminars for health care professionals and pump users.

By sensitizing the pump user to subtle warning cues for hypoglycemia, BGAT helps increase the likelihood that he or she will test blood glucose and take appropriate action at the earliest sign of possible hypoglycemia.

The diary is the most important learning component of blood glucose awareness training. It allows the participant to practice estimating his or her blood glucose level based on relevant cues and to receive immediate feedback on the accuracy of the estimate. Several times each day, participants complete a diary entry just prior to self-monitoring of blood glucose. This requires the individual to:

1. Scan himself for blood glucose-related information, taking into consideration internal cues, as well as other glucose-relevant factors (e.g., recent food intake);

2. Estimate the blood glucose level on the basis of these cues;

3. Measure and record the actual blood glucose value, and finally;

4. Evaluate the accuracy of the estimate.

During weekly sessions, participants in the BGAT program systematically review their blood glucose diaries for hypoglycemic entries. For those hypoglycemic levels that were successfully detected, participants attempt to elucidate the internal and/or external cues that were helpful in making an accurate estimate. For hypoglycemia that went undetected, they try to determine what cues may have been missed, misinterpreted, or relied upon in error. The use of incorrect cues is a common reason for poor detection of low blood glucose (e.g., "I had recently eaten, so I knew that my blood glucose couldn't be low"). Common patterns of errors include: consistent overestimation or underestimation of actual blood glucose levels, overdependence on external or internal cues, and inability to detect low blood glucose during busy work hours.

Through regular examination of blood glucose diaries, BGAT participants learn to identify reliable symptoms of hypoglycemia and to distinguish those cues that are predictive from those that are misleading. For example, one individual, employed as a carpenter, knew that if he dropped several nails in a row, he should consider the possibility of hypoglycemia and check his blood glucose level. Another participant recognized that not attempting to hit the tennis ball at his appropriate turn during a doubles match signaled the need to check his blood glucose.

People who have taken BGAT generally improve in their ability to recognize and treat low blood glucose levels. Even individuals without reduced awareness find blood glucose awareness training useful in decreasing the frequency of low blood glucose episodes. Before training, hypoglycemia may be recognized only about 50 percent of the time; after training nearly 75 percent of hypoglycemic episodes are recognized (44,45). BGAT has also been shown to reduce the frequency of severe hypoglycemia and motor vehicle violations over a one-year period, without compromising glycemic control (45). A four-year follow-up study links BGAT to a significant decrease in automobile accidents (46).

Blood glucose awareness training provides an extremely useful tool to the person using CSII. By sensitizing the pump user to subtle warning cues for hypoglycemia, BGAT helps increase the likelihood that he or she will test blood glucose and take appropriate action at the earliest sign of possible hypoglycemia. Blood glucose awareness training can help pump users achieve desired levels of glycemic control with enhanced safety and confidence.

SUMMARY

Hypoglycemia is a risk for people using insulin, and the risk for severe hypoglycemia increases as blood glucose target goals approach normal levels. The insulin pump offers pharmacokinetic advantages that can reduce the risk of hypoglycemia during intensified therapy. Appropriate individualization of blood glucose target levels is critical in helping patients to avoid severe hypoglycemia, as is thorough training in the recognition and treatment of even mild hypoglycemia.

REFERENCES

1. The Diabetes Control and Complications Trial Research Group. The effect of intensive treatment of diabetes on the development and progression of long-term complications in insulin-dependent diabetes mellitus. *N Engl J Med* 1993;329:977-986.

2. White NH. Hypoglycemia: a limiting factor in implementing intensive therapy. *Clinical Diabetes* 1994;12:101-105.

3. Bode B, Steed D, Davidson P. Long-term pump use and SMBG in 205 patients. *Diabetes* 1994;43(Suppl 1):220A.

4. Ronn B, Mathiesen ER, Vang L, Lorup B, Deckert T. Evaluation of insulin pump treatment under routine conditions. *Diabetes Res Clin Pract* 1989;3:191-196.

5. Chantelau E, Spraul M, Muhlhauser I, Gause R, Berger M. Long term safety, efficacy and side-effects of continuous subcutaneous insulin infusion treatment for type 1 (insulin dependent) diabetes mellitus: a one centre experience. *Diabetologia* 1989;32:421-426.

6. Wredling R, Lins PE, Adamson U. Factors influencing the clinical outcome of continuous subcutaneous insulin infusion in routine practice. *Diabetes Res Clin Pract* 1993;19:59-67.

7. Eichner HL, Selam JL, Holleman CB, Worcester BR, Turner DS, Charles MA. Reduction of severe hypoglycemic events in type I (insulin dependent) diabetic patients using continuous subcutaneous insulin infusion. *Diabetes Res* 1998;8:189-193.

8. Bell DSH, Cutter G, Clements RS. The feasibility of long-term treatment of diabetes with continuous subcutaneous insulin infusion. *Diab Nutr Metab* 1993;6:57-60.

9. Hirsch IB, Farkas-Hirsch R, Cryer PE. Continuous subcutaneous insulin infusion for the treatment of diabetic patients with hypoglycemia unawareness. *Diab Nutr Metab* 1991;4:41-43.

10. Towler DA, Havlin CD, Craft S, Cryer PE. Mechanisms of awareness of hypoglycemia: perception of neurogenic (predominantly cholinergic) rather than neuroglycopenic symptoms. *Diabetes* 1993;42:1791-1798.

11. Cryer PE, Fisher JN, Shamoon. Hypoglycemia. *Diabetes Care* 1994;17:734-748.

12. Frier BM. Hypoglycaemia and diabetes. *Diabet Med* 1986;3:513-525.

13. Cox D, Gonder-Frederick L, Clarke W. Driving decrements in type I diabetes during moderate hypoglycemia. *Diabetes* 1993;42:239-243.

14. Deary IJ, Crawford JR, Hepburn DA, Langan SJ, Blackmore LM, Frier BM. Severe hypoglycemia and intelligence in adult patients with insulin-treated diabetes. *Diabetes* 1993;42:341-344.

15. Wredling R, Levander S, Adamson U, Pins PE. Permanent neuropsychological impairment after recurrent episodes of severe hypoglycemia in man. *Diabetologia* 1990;33:152-157.

16. Reichard P, Britz A, Rosenqvist U. Intensified conventional insulin treatment and neuropsychological impairment. *Br Med J* 1991;303:1439-1442.

17. Deary IJ, Frier BM. Intensified conventional insulin treatment and neuropsychological impairment (Letter). *Br Med J* 1992;304:447

18. Golden MP, Ingersoll GM, Brack CJ, Russell BA, Wright JC, Hyberty TJ. Longitudinal relationship of asymptomatic hypoglycemia to cognitive function in IDDM. *Diabetes Care* 1989;12:89-93.

19. Santiago JV, Levandoski LA, Bubb J. Hypoglycemia in patients with type I diabetes. In: Lebovitz HE, ed. *Therapy for Diabetes Mellitus and Related Disorders*, Second Edition. Alexandria, VA: American Diabetes Association; 1994, 170-177.

20. Bendtson I. Nocturnal hypoglycaemia. In: Federlin K, Keen H, Mehnert H., eds. *Hypoglycaemia and Human Insulin*. New York, NY: Georg Thieme Verlag Stuttgart; 1991:39-42.

21. Hirsch IB, Heller SR, Cryer PE. Increased symptoms of hypoglycaemia in the standing position in insulin-dependent diabetes mellitus. *Clinical Science* 1991;80:583-586.

22. Bolli GB, Perriello G, Fanelli CG, DePeo P. Nocturnal blood glucose control in type I diabetes mellitus. *Diabetes Care* 1993;16(Suppl 3):71-89.

23. Puczynski S, Puczynski M. Commentary on epidemiology of severe hypoglycemia in the Diabetes Control and Complications Trial. *Diabetes Spectrum* 1994;7:243-244.

24. Cox D, Gonder-Frederick L, Antoun B, Cryer P, Clarke WL. Psychobehavioral metabolic parameters of severe hypoglycemic episodes. *Diabetes Care* 1990;13:458-459.

25. The DCCT Research Group. Epidemiology of severe hypoglycemia in the Diabetes Control and Complications Trial. *Am Journal of Med* 1991;90:450-459.

26. The DCCT Research Group. Implementation of treatment protocols in the Diabetes Control and Complications Trial. *Diabetes Care* 1995;18:361-376.

27. Mecklenburg RS, Benson EA, Benson JW, Fredlund PN, Guinn T, Metz RJ, Nielsen RL, Sannar CA. Acute complications associated with insulin infusion pump therapy. Report of experience with 161 patients. JAMA 1984;252:3265-3269.

28. Lauritzen T, Pramming S, Deckert T, Binder C. Pharmacokinetics of continuous subcutaneous insulin infusion. *Diabetologia* 1983;24:326-329.

29. Havlin CE, Cryer PE. Nocturnal hypoglycemia does not commonly result in major morning hypoglycemia in patients with diabetes mellitus. *Diabetes Care* 1987;10:141-147.

30. Dagogo-Jack A, Chatchalit R, Cryer PE. Reversal of hypoglycemia unawareness, but not of defective glucose counterregulation, in IDDM. *Diabetes* 1994;43:1426-1434.

31. Cryer PE. Hypoglycemia begets hypoglycemia in IDDM. *Diabetes* 1993;42:1691-1693.

32. MacLeod KM, Gold AE, Frier BM. Frequency of severe hypoglycemia in insulin-dependent diabetic patients with altered awareness of hypoglycemia (ABS). *Diabetes* 1993;42:26A.

33. Fanelli CG, Epifano L, Rambotti M, Pampaneli S, Di Vincenzo A, Modarelli F, Lepore M, Annibale B, Ciofetta M, Bottini P, Pordellati F, Scionti L, Santeusanio F, Brunetti P, Bolli GB. Meticulous prevention of hypoglycemia normalizes the glycemic threshold and magnitude of most of neuroendocrine responses to, symptoms of, and cognitive function during hypoglycemia in intensively treated patients with short term IDDM. *Diabetes* 1993;42:l683-l689.

34. Fanelli C, Pampanelli S, Epifano L, Rambotti AM, Di Vencenso A, Modarelli F, Ciofetta M, Lepore M, Annibale B, Torlone E, Perriello G, De Feo P, Santeusanio F, Brunetti P, Bolli GB. Long-term recovery from unawareness, deficient counterregulation and lack of cognitive dysfunction during hypoglycaemia, following institution of rational, intensive insulin therapy in IDDM. *Diabetologia* 1994;37:1265-1276.

35. Hoeldtke RD, Boden G. Epinephrine secretion, hypoglycemia unawareness, and diabetic autonomic neuropathy. *Ann Intern Med* 1994;120:512-517.

36. Cryer PE. Iatrogenic hypoglycemia as a cause of hypoglycemia-associated autonomic failure in IDDM: a vicious cycle. *Diabetes* 1992;41:255-260.

37. Cox DJ, Gonder-Frederick LA, Polonsky W, Schlundt D, Kovatchev B, Clarke WL. Recent hypoglycemia influences the probability of subsequent hypoglycemia in type I patients. *Diabetes* 1993;42(Suppl 1):126A.

38. Gold AE, MacLeod KM, Frier BM. Frequency of severe hypoglycemia in patients with type I diabetes with impaired awareness of hypoglycemia. *Diabetes Care* 1994;17:697-703.

39. Heller SR, Cryer PE. Reduced neuroendocrine and symptomatic responses to subsequent hypoglycemia after one episode of hypoglycemia in nondiabetic humans. *Diabetes* 1991;40:223-226

40. Dagogo-Jack SE, Craft SM, Cryer PE. Hypoglycemia-associated autonomic failure in insulin-dependent diabetes mellitus. Recent antecedent hypoglycemia reduces autonomic responses to, symptoms of, and defense against subsequent hypoglycemia. *J Clin Invest* 1993;91:819-828.

41. Hirsch IB, Boyle PJ, Craft S, Cryer PE. Higher glycemic thresholds for symptoms during B-adrenergic blockade in IDDM. *Diabetes* 1991;40:1177-1188.

42. Cox DJ, Gonder-Frederick LA, Lee JH, Julian D, Clarke WL. Blood glucose awareness training among patients with IDDM: effects and correlates. *Diabetes Care* 1989;12:313-318.

43. Cox DJ, Gonder-Frederick LA, Polonsky W, Schlundt D, Julian D, Clarke WL. A multicenter evaluation of blood glucose awareness training II. *Diabetes Care* 1995;18:523-528.

44. Cox W, Gonder-Frederick LA, Julian D, Cryer P. Intensive versus standard blood glucose awareness training (BGAT) with insulin-dependent diabetes: Mechanisms and ancillary effects. *Psychosom Med* 1991;53:453-462.

45. Cox DJ, Gonder-Frederick LA, Kovatchev B, Polonsky W, Schlundt D, Clarke WL. Reduction of severe hypoglycemia with blood glucose awareness training (BGAT-2). *Diabetes* 1995;44(Suppl 1):27A.

46. Cox DJ, Gonder-Frederick LA, Julian D, Clarke W. Long-term follow-up evaluation of blood glucose awareness training. *Diabetes Care* 1994;17:1-5.

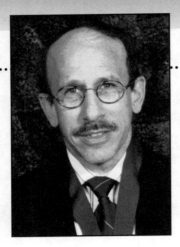

ANDREW J. DREXLER, MD, FACE

Andrew Jay Drexler, MD, is a diabetologist in New York City and a faculty member of the New York University School of Medicine. He is chairman of the Medical Advisory Committee of the New York Chapter of the Juvenile Diabetes Foundation and a past chairman of the Clinical Society of the New York Downstate Affiliate of the American Diabetes Association. He has been working with insulin pumps and in the field of diabetes and pregnancy for the past 15 years.

PUMP THERAPY IN PRECONCEPTION AND PREGNANCY 13

The goal of insulin therapy in managing diabetes during pregnancy is to maintain blood glucose levels as near normal as possible. Use of an insulin pump provides a simple, convenient means for the intensification of insulin therapy needed to achieve this level of control. The purpose of this chapter is to highlight the benefits and techniques of using continuous subcutaneous insulin infusion (CSII) to provide the stringent glycemic control necessary to improve the quality of the pregnancy and reduce risks to the fetus.

OPTIMIZING GLYCEMIC CONTROL

During pregnancy, blood glucose levels are normally lower, even for women who do not have diabetes. Glucose goals for a pregnant woman with diabetes must be set at these physiologic levels and be strictly controlled in order to provide the environment required for a successful pregnancy that produces a healthy baby. Strict blood glucose control means keeping blood glucose levels as near normal as possible. Recommended glucose target levels in pregnancy are shown in Table 1.

Elevated blood glucose levels during embryogenesis (two to eight weeks' gestation) are associated with serious congenital anomalies (1), while elevated levels in the second and third trimesters are more likely to result in fetal complications such as:

1. Intrauterine growth delay (2)

2. Macrosomia, or a birth weight of greater than nine pounds (3,4)

IN THIS CHAPTER

Preconception Care

Insulin Requirements

Basal, Bolus and Food Adjustments

Risks and Complications

The physiologic delivery of regular insulin by a pump and its more predictable absorption can help reduce the incidence of hypoglycemia, which potentiates the nausea and vomiting during early pregnancy.

3. Neonatal hypoglycemia (3,5)

4. Respiratory distress syndrome (6)

5. Erythema (3)

6. Hyperbilirubinemia (3,5)

Intensified maternal glycemic control and maintenance of normal glycemic levels throughout pregnancy have been shown to be paramount in reducing the incidence of such complications (7-9).

For the mother, the physiologic delivery of regular insulin by a pump and its more predictable absorption can help reduce the incidence of hypoglycemia, which potentiates the nausea and vomiting during early pregnancy (10,11). It can also reduce the risk of nocturnal hypoglycemia, which is likely to occur as a result of the continuous consumption of glucose throughout the night by the fetus (1). CSII is helpful in decreasing the wide blood glucose variations and postprandial hyperglycemia common in pregnancy (12).

Table 1

Suggested Target Blood Glucose Ranges in Pregnancy [1,3,24]

Fasting (before breakfast)	60-90 mg/dL
Before lunch, supper and bedtime snack	60-90 mg/dL
1 hour postprandial	120-140 mg/dL
2 AM - 6 PM	>60 mg/dL

Glycosylated hemoglobin levels should be within the normal range for the individual laboratory.

PRECONCEPTION CARE

Pregnancy for a woman with diabetes requires careful consideration and planning by both prospective parents. Once the decision to become pregnant has been made, the woman, her partner, and the health care team should work together to develop an individualized pregnancy management program. During the preconception period, the health care team should gather baseline data for perinatal risks. The following clinical factors should be included in preconception visits (13):

1. An assessment of glycemic control by means of glycated hemoglobin (HbA$_{1c}$) values, as well as current postmeal blood glucose levels.

2. An ophthalmologic examination to assess the status of any retinopathy.

3. A 24-hour urine collection for creatinine clearance, total proteinuria and microalbuminuria to assess any preexistent or developing nephropathy.

4. A review of the diet.

5. A review of any current exercise program.

The prospective parents should be instructed in the importance of strict blood glucose control before and during pregnancy. In order to ensure the best possible outcome, prepregnancy blood glucose goals should be the same as those required for optimal glycemic control in nonpregnant individuals (see Chapter 5, *Establishing & Verifying Basal Rates*). Ideally, normal blood glucose levels should be achieved and maintained for at least three months prior to conception.

It is also important to address the psychological well-being of the patient and her partner during prepregnancy visits. For example, pregnancy may cause discomfort with the body image, and wearing a pump can add to these feelings. This and other concerns the patient or her partner may have regarding pump use and pregnancy should be addressed early in the process.

Initiation of Pump Therapy During Pregnancy

While it is ideal to initiate pump therapy during preconception, it can be successfully initiated in the pregnant woman. In this case, inpatient initiation is preferable to ensure that counseling factors are addressed and that all necessary self-management skills are in place. (Refer to Chapter 4, *Initiating Pump Therapy*, for details of inpatient initiation.)

INSULIN REQUIREMENTS DURING PREGNANCY

Pregnancy is a condition associated with constant change, not the least of which is a continual change in insulin requirements. For instance, during the first trimester, when nausea and vomiting may occur and nocturnal hypoglycemia is likely, insulin doses may actually need to be reduced. As pregnancy progresses, the placenta secretes increased levels of insulin-antagonistic hormones such as estrogen, progesterone and human placental lactogen, resulting in an increased insulin requirement. Increased hormone levels can cause a woman's insulin requirement to double by the end of pregnancy (14).

The degree of increase in the insulin need at any stage in gestation varies considerably from woman to woman (15). A pregnant woman with diabetes needs to be reassured that an increase in her insulin requirement is normal and

Normal blood glucose levels should be achieved and maintained for at least three months prior to conception.

expected, and is an indication that her baby is growing. Typical changes in the total daily insulin requirement over the course of a pregnancy are summarized in Table 2.

Table 2

Estimated Total Daily Insulin Requirements

Stage	U/kg current body weight
Prepregnancy	0.6
Weeks 6-18 Gestation	0.7
Weeks 18-26 Gestation	0.8
Weeks 26-36 Gestation	0.9
Weeks 36-Delivery	1.0
Postpartum	<0.6

Basal rates and bolus doses may need to be changed every few days as determined by blood glucose measurements.

It must be emphasized that exact insulin doses **cannot be assumed** at any stage in gestation. Insulin requirements are determined solely on the basis of blood glucose levels, making rigorous self-monitoring of blood glucose critical in assessing and maintaining control. It is strongly recommended that a pregnant woman with diabetes check and record her blood glucose **at least 8 times per day:** before meals, one hour after meals, at bedtime and at least once during the night (2 AM to 3 AM). Checking blood glucose levels postprandially may be a new concept for the woman with diabetes. She should be instructed in the appropriate times for testing and be supplied with appropriate recordkeeping forms. The one-hour postprandial blood glucose level represents the highest blood glucose level after the meal and can be valuable in helping the woman anticipate hypoglycemia (16). If the one-hour postprandial blood glucose level is in the lower end of the target range, the chance of subsequent hypoglycemia is increased.

Basal and Bolus Adjustments
Using a pump is a highly efficient means of managing insulin dosing changes and adjustments (17,18). For example, an increase in the early morning basal rate is beneficial in managing a dawn phenomenon, and a decrease in the night-time basal rate may be helpful in counteracting nocturnal hypoglycemia. Basal rates and bolus doses may need to be changed every few days as determined by blood glucose measurements. General guidelines for adjusting basal rates and

boluses in the pregnant woman are as follows:

1. If the one-hour postprandial blood glucose level is acceptable but the next premeal blood glucose is above target range, the basal rate should be increased.

2. If the one-hour postprandial blood glucose is ≥40 mg/dL above the premeal level, the woman should take supplemental insulin and increase the premeal bolus for the same meal on the next and subsequent days.

3. If the one-hour postprandial blood glucose is less than the premeal level, the premeal bolus for that meal should be decreased on the next and subsequent days.

4. If the woman is unable to eat due to nausea, the basal rate(s) covers her insulin requirement and protects against hypoglycemia. If she can tolerate food, she may give a small bolus (perhaps 0.5 unit) when she sits down to eat and take additional insulin as she eats more food. This way, if she becomes nauseous after beginning to eat, she can discontinue further bolusing without fear of having taken too much insulin for an anticipated meal.

5. If the premeal blood glucose level is within target range, the woman should give the entire bolus 30 minutes before eating. If the premeal blood glucose is elevated, she should give the bolus plus supplemental insulin and wait until her blood glucose is below 100 mg/dL before eating. This requires that she check her blood glucose every 20 minutes after giving the bolus.

Adjustments such as these are necessary to accommodate changes in the woman's insulin sensitivity and must be made on an individualized basis.

Detailed information regarding basal and bolus adjustments and supplemental insulin doses can be found in Chapters 5 and 6. A pregnant woman should be instructed to keep meticulous records of all blood glucose readings and to communicate with the diabetes team at least once every other day. Insulin requirements should be reviewed by the woman and her health care team at least once a week to ensure that approximately 40 percent of her total daily dose is basal insulin and the remaining 60 percent comes from bolus and supplemental insulin doses. This protocol allows for early identification of undesirable blood glucose patterns and initiation of appropriate insulin adjustments.

FOOD INTAKE ADJUSTMENTS AND MEAL PLANNING

The daily nutritional needs of a pregnant woman with diabetes are the same as those of a nondiabetic pregnant woman. A meal plan assessment by a dietitian can help determine if nutritional needs are being met. Blood glucose measurements, urine ketones, appetite, and weight gain should all be considered in developing and evaluating an individualized meal plan that will promote optimal blood glucose control.

A nutritionally appropriate diet comprised of 40 percent carbohydrate is recommended and should be individualized to meet the woman's daily caloric needs. A meal plan that distributes the total daily carbohydrate intake over three meals and three to four snacks helps to minimize blood glucose variations and facilitate tighter glycemic control. The flexibility provided by an insulin pump greatly simplifies the handling of the multiple boluses required by such a plan.

One such approach to carbohydrate distribution is the so-called "Rule of Eighteenths" (3). This method requires the woman, with the help of her dietitian, to estimate her usual total daily carbohydrate intake and then calculate the portions of carbohydrate for each meal or snack. For example, suppose a woman's total daily carbohydrate intake is 200 grams. This total is divided by 18, which gives approximately 11 grams per "eighteenth." These 11-gram portions are distributed over the day's meals and snacks as shown in Table 3. At breakfast, for example, the woman should eat 2/18 of the day's total carbohydrate, in this case 2 x 11 grams = 22 grams.

In typical meal plans, the breakfast carbohydrate is very small when compared to lunch and dinner. Most people tend to be more insulin-resistant in the morning, which results in an increase in the insulin required to yield an acceptable

---

Table 3

"THE RULE OF EIGHTEENTHS"

Meal/Snack	Portion of Total Carbohydrate
Breakfast	2/18
Midmorning Snack	1/18
Lunch	5/18
Midafternoon Snack	1/18
Dinner	6/18
After Dinner Snack	1/18
Bedtime Snack	2/18

The calculation of this diet is based on the formula of 30 kcal/kg body weight (40% carbohydrate, 20% protein and 40% fat)

one-hour postprandial blood glucose level. Pregnant women with diabetes often do best when they avoid foods containing simple sugars, such as fruits or juices, at the breakfast meal, as such foods cause the blood glucose level to rise at a rate that is hard to match with insulin.

The continuous drain on maternal glucose stores by the fetus makes eating snacks a necessity. A pregnant woman with diabetes whose basal rate(s) is correct and whose postprandial blood glucose levels are within target range still must eat between-meal and bedtime snacks to reduce the risk of hypoglycemic episodes (11). However, if blood glucose is >120 one hour after the meal, the blood glucose should be tested before the snack and the snack witheld if the blood glucose is still >120 mg/dL.

SITE SELECTION AND SKIN IRRITATION

As pregnancy advances, abdominal sites for infusion become less comfortable due to the skin stretching that is necessary to make way for an enlarging uterus. Alternative sites include the upper arm, upper outer thighs and upper outer buttocks. No matter which site is chosen, the woman should make sure that the skin at the site can be "pinched up" before attempting insertion of the infusion set.

During pregnancy, the skin has a tendency toward dryness, which may increase the incidence of skin irritation, particularly at the infusion site. Use of an antibacterial cleanser, such as Hibiclens, may reduce skin irritation and is preferable to alcohol for cleansing the skin prior to inserting the infusion set. Use of a soft teflon cannula, such as the Sof-set™ by MiniMed, can also help to reduce skin and site irritation.

LABOR AND DELIVERY

The onset of labor brings about changes in the insulin requirement, and in some situations, the mode of insulin delivery. During active labor, insulin requirements decrease dramatically. If the pump is left in place when the woman is in active labor, the basal rate is typically set at a very low level (e.g., 0.1 to 0.2 unit per hour). However, the basal rate will vary with the strength of the labor. Caloric needs during labor are met by an intravenous infusion of glucose. In situations where it is not possible to leave the pump in place, a second IV line is started for insulin administration.

The goal of metabolic management during labor is to maintain maternal blood glucose levels at 60 to 100 mg/dL. Blood glucose testing should be done hourly so that appropriate adjustments in the basal rate or glucose infusion can be made in order to achieve this range (19). Because blood glucose values in excess of 120 mg/dL stimulate insulin production in the baby, which can result in neonatal hypoglycemia shortly after birth (3), they should be quickly treated with insulin boluses via the pump or the IV insulin line.

With delivery and the removal of the placenta, the level of chorionic somatomammotropin (human placental lactogen) and its effect on insulin resistance rapidly subside, which can further reduce the insulin requirement.

POSTPARTUM CONSIDERATIONS

In the immediate postpartum period, insulin requirements are usually lower than those during prepregnancy. If delivery was by cesarean section, basal insulin may be all the woman requires for the first two or three postoperative days, as calorie intake is normally limited following surgery. Regardless of the means of delivery, adjustment of insulin needs in the postpartum period should be individualized based on SMBG results. These adjustments are easily managed with the use of an insulin pump.

The birth of a baby adds an entirely new dimension to daily routines. The use of an insulin pump helps provide the flexibility the mother needs to adapt to new schedules and can help her maintain a sense of well-being and control of her diabetes in this time of readjustment. If the mother chooses to breastfeed, which is encouraged, her insulin requirement will generally be less (14). Specifically, the overnight basal requirement may be markedly reduced due to siphoning of glucose into the milk fed to the baby in the middle of the night.

RISKS AND COMPLICATIONS ASSOCIATED WITH PUMP THERAPY IN PREGNANCY

Diabetic Ketoacidosis

The main risk associated with pump therapy in pregnancy is diabetic ketoacidosis (DKA). The increased insulin demand, rising levels of counterregulatory hormones, and continually increasing rate of fetal glucose consumption that occur in pregnancy all heighten the risk for developing ketoacidosis. DKA has a fetal mortality rate of approximately 50 percent (20), so even a brief interruption of insulin delivery must be avoided at all costs. Therefore, a pregnant woman who is using CSII should be especially cautious that her pump and infusion set are working properly.

The following methods for avoiding hyperglycemia are a critical part of the pregnant pump user's self-help skills:

- Frequent blood glucose monitoring should be used to prevent undetected interruption of insulin delivery.
- The infusion set MUST be changed every 24 hours or more frequently during pregnancy and **always** when an unexplained high blood glucose level occurs.
- If the blood glucose is >160 mg/dL, supplemental insulin should be given immediately by injection instead of by pump. Detailed guidelines for preventing DKA are presented in Chapter 11, *DKA Prevention.*

- Urine ketones should be checked every morning and whenever the blood glucose is above the target level. If ketones are positive, the physician should be notified immediately.

To avoid the risk of DKA developing overnight due to an absorption problem or pump failure, some clinicians recommend adding an injection of NPH or Lente insulin at bedtime to work concurrently with a reduced basal rate provided by the pump. However, a more aggressive approach to reducing the risk of overnight DKA is to require the woman to check her blood glucose at least twice during the night (2 AM and 5 AM) and take supplemental insulin if necessary. This extra, overnight testing is also helpful in detecting any problem with the pump that might result in interrupted insulin delivery and DKA (e.g., a dislodged infusion set).

A Worsening of Vascular Complications

Retinopathy and nephropathy are known to worsen with the onset of intensive insulin therapy, and to reverse with time (21-23). With pregnancy, there may be increased deterioration of these conditions. The degree to which these conditions advance is directly related to how rapidly normal glycemia is established, thus emphasizing the need for achieving strict control **prior to conception**. These conditions also tend to reverse after the birth of the baby.

SUMMARY AND CONCLUSIONS

Early education and counseling of a woman with diabetes who wishes to become pregnant are essential to ensuring a successful pregnancy. Meticulous glycemic control before conception and during gestation significantly reduces the risk of congenital anomalies and neonatal complications. For the woman who is already pregnant, achieving near-normal glycemia as soon as possible improves the probability of a successful pregnancy.

Use of an insulin pump provides a simple, efficient and effective way to achieve the required level of glycemic control to satisfy each of these needs.

REFERENCES

1. Santiago JV, ed. Pregnancy. In: *Medical Management of Insulin Dependent Type I Diabetes*, Second Edition. Alexandria, VA: American Diabetes Association; 1994:90-98.

2. Pedersen JF, Molsted-Pedersen L. Early growth retardation in diabetic pregnancy. In: Jovanovic L, Peterson CM, Fuhrmann K, eds. *Diabetes and Pregnancy*, First Edition. New York, NY: Praeger, 1986.

3. Jovanovic L, Druzin M, Peterson CM. Effect of euglycemia on the outcome of pregnancy in insulin-dependent diabetic women as compared with normal control subjects. *Am J Med* 1981;71:921-927.

4. Dandona P, Boag F, Fonesca V, Menon RK. Correspondence: diabetes and pregnancy. *N Engl J Med* 1986;314:58-60.

5. Ylinen K, Raivio K, Teramo K. Haemoglobin A1c predicts the perinatal outcome in insulin-dependent diabetic pregnancies. *Brit J Obstet Gynecol* 1981;88:961-967.

6. Fadel H, Saad SA, Nelson GH, Davis HC. Effect of maternal-fetal disorders on lung maturation: I. Diabetes Mellitus. *Am J Obstet Gynecol* 1986;155:544-553.

7. Reece AS, Homko C. Management of pregnant women with diabetes. In: Lebovitz HE, ed. *Therapy for Diabetes Mellitus and Related Disorders*, Second Edition. Alexandria, VA: American Diabetes Association; 1994:17-24.

8. Kitzmiller JL, Gavin LA, Gin GD, Jovanovic-Peterson L, Main EK, Zigrang WD. Preconception care of diabetes glycemic control prevents congenital anomalies. *JAMA* 1991;265:731-736.

9. Rosenn B, Miodovnik M, St. John DP, Siddiqi TA, Khoury J, Mimouni F. Minor congenital malformations in infants of insulin-dependent diabetic women: association with poor glycemic control. *Obstet Gynecol* 1990;76:745-749.

10. Binder C, Lauritzen T, Faber O, Pramming S. Insulin pharmacokinetics. *Diabetes Care* 1984;7:188-200.

11. Kitzmiller JL, Younger AD, Hare JW, Phillippe M, Vignati L, Fargnoli B, Grause A. Continuous subcutaneous insulin therapy during early pregnancy. *Obstet Gynecol* 1985;66:606-611.

12. Blumenthal AS, Abdul KRW. Review: Diagnosis, classification, and metabolic management of diabetes in pregnancy: therapeutic impact of self-monitoring of blood glucose and of newer methods of insulin delivery. *Obstet Gynecol Survey* 1987;42:593-604.

13. Abrams RS. Pre-pregnancy counseling for women with diabetes. *Practical Diabetology* 1990;7:1-3.

14. Hollander P, Pratt L. Pregnancy and diabetes: careful planning and control. In: Franz MJ, ed. *Learning to Live Well with Diabetes*. Minneapolis, MN: DCI Publishing; 1991:349-361.

15. Steel JM, Johnstone FD, Hume R, Mao J-H. Insulin requirements during pregnancy in women with type I diabetes. *Obstet Gynecol* 1994;83:253-258.

16. Peterson CM, Jovanovic L, Brownlee M, Cerami A. Closing the loop, practical and theoretical. *Diabetes Care* 1980;3:318-323.

17. Rudolf M, Coustan D, Sherwin RS, Bates SE, Felig P, Genel M, Tamborlane WV. Efficacy of the insulin pump in the home treatment of pregnant diabetics. *Diabetes* 1981;30:891-895.

18. Potter JM, Reckless JPD, Cullen DR. Effect of subcutaneous insulin infusion and conventional regimes on 24-hour variations of blood glucose and intermediary metabolites in the third trimester of diabetic pregnancy. *Diabetologia* 1981;21:534-540.

19. Rossi G, Diamond MP. Antepartum and intrapartum obstetric care. In: Lebovitz HE, ed. *Therapy for Diabetes Mellitus and Related Disorders.* Alexandria, VA: American Diabetes Association; 1994:25-31.

20. Kitzmiller JL. Diabetic ketoacidosis and pregnancy. In: Queenan JT, ed. *Managing OB-Gyn Emergencies*, Second Edition. Oradell NJ: Medical Economics; 1983:44-55.

21. Diabetes Control and Complications Trial Research Group (DCCT). The effect of intensive treatment of diabetes on the development and progression of long-term complications in insulin dependent diabetes mellitus. *N Engl J Med* 1993;329:977-986.

22. Kroc Collaborative Group. Diabetic retinopathy after two years of intensified insulin treatment; follow-up of the Kroc Collaborative Study. *JAMA* 1988;260:37-40.

23. Lauritzen T, Frost-Larsen K, Larsen HW, Deckert T, Steno Study Group. Two years' experience with continuous subcutaneous insulin infusion in relation to retinopathy and neuropathy. *Diabetes* 1985;34(Suppl 3):74-79.

24. Jovanovic L, Peterson CM, Saxena BB, Dawood MY, Saudek CD. Feasibility of maintaining normal glucose profiles in insulin-dependent pregnant diabetic women. *Am J Med* 1980;68:105-112.

INDEX

NOTES

NOTES